Chemical Peels in Clinical Practice

This book has been written with the aim of making a practitioner's peeling experience easier and more practical. It contains sample patient forms, over 250 illustrations, and a wealth of tips for patient guidance and safe clinical practice.

Series in Cosmetic and Laser Therapy

About the Series

The world of cosmetic and aesthetic medicine and surgery has grown greatly in size and complexity over recent years, and the series in *Cosmetic and Laser Therapy* keeps readers up to date with the latest clinical therapies to improve and rejuvenate the appearance of skin, hair, and nails. Published in association with the *Journal of Cosmetic and Laser Therapy*, each volume in the series is prepared separately and typically focuses on a topical theme. Volumes are published on an occasional basis, according to the emergence of new developments.

Handbook of Cosmetic Skin Care, Second Edition
Avi Shai, Howard I. Maibach, Robert Baran

Cosmetic Bootcamp Primer: Comprehensive Aesthetic Management
Kenneth Beer, Mary P. Lupo, Vic A. Narurkar

Illustrated Manual of Injectable Fillers: A Technical Guide to the Volumetric Approach to Whole Body Rejuvenation, First Edition
Neil S. Sadick, Paul J. Carniol, Deborshi Roy, Luitgard Wiest

Comprehensive Aesthetic Rejuvenation: A Regional Approach
Jenny Kim, Gary Lask, Andrew Nelson

Textbook of Chemical Peels: Superficial, Medium, and Deep Peels in Cosmetic Practice, Second Edition
Philippe Deprez, Philippe Deprez

Textbook of Cosmetic Dermatology, Fifth Edition
Robert Baran, Howard I. Maibach

Disorders of Fat and Cellulite: Advances in Diagnosis and Treatment
David J. Goldberg, Alexander L. Berlin

Botulinum Toxins in Clinical Aesthetic Practice 3E, Volume Two: Functional Anatomy and Injection Techniques
Anthony V Benedetto

Botulinum Toxins in Clinical Aesthetic Practice 3E, Volume One: Clinical Adaptations
Anthony V Benedetto

Botulinum Toxins in Clinical Aesthetic Practice 3E: Two Volume Set
Anthony V Benedetto

Aesthetic Rejuvenation Challenges and Solutions: A World Perspective
Paul J. Carniol, Gary D. Monheit

Illustrated Manual of Injectable Fillers, Second Edition
Neil S. Sadick

Adapting Dermal Fillers in Clinical Practice
Yates Yen-Yu Chao, Sebastian Cotofana

Cosmeceutical Science in Clinical Practice, Second Edition
Neil S Sadick, Mary P Lupo, and Zoe Diana Draelos

Chemical Peels in Clinical Practice: A Practical Guide to Superficial, Medium, and Deep Peels
Xavier Goodarzian

For more information about this series please visit: https://www.crcpress.com/Series-in-Cosmetic-and-Laser-Therapy/book-series/CRCCOSLASTHE

Chemical Peels in Clinical Practice

A Practical Guide to Superficial, Medium, and Deep Peels

Xavier G Goodarzian

MD(Hons), MRCGP, PGDiplClinDerm, PGCertCosMed, MBCAM
Medical Director, Dr Xavier Clinic
Southampton and London, United Kingdom

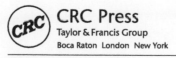

CRC Press
Taylor & Francis Group
Boca Raton London New York

CRC Press is an imprint of the
Taylor & Francis Group, an **informa** business

Designed cover image: Xavier Goodarzian

First edition published 2024
by CRC Press
6000 Broken Sound Parkway NW, Suite 300, Boca Raton, FL 33487-2742

and by CRC Press
4 Park Square, Milton Park, Abingdon, Oxon, OX14 4RN

CRC Press is an imprint of Taylor & Francis Group, LLC

© 2024 Xavier Goodarzian

ISBN: 9781032154282 (hbk)
ISBN: 9781032154329 (pbk)
ISBN: 9781003244134 (ebk)

DOI: 10.1201/9781003244134

Typeset in Times
by Deanta Global Publishing Services, Chennai, India

Contents

Preface

Thank you for purchasing this book. I hope it gives you some inspiration and practical guidance to build chemical peels in your treatment portfolio.

For me personally, chemical peels were one of the reasons I actually ended up pursuing a career in aesthetic medicine. I started my medical degree in Belgium in 1993 and at some point during my studies I came across a textbook in the library about cosmetic dermatology. Within that book there was a chapter about skin resurfacing with chemical peels, and I was so inspired by that book that I then decided I wanted to do something related to skin as a doctor. Later on towards the end of my medical studies I spent six months working at the dermatology department in the hospital as a Junior Doctor, and I wrote a dissertation on skin ageing and active ingredients in skincare. So it is fair to say that I was fascinated by skin rejuvenation and almost obsessed with subjects such as active skincare ingredients and chemical peels from early on.

In 2005 I did my first training in chemical peels, and I learnt how to perform superficial AHA peels. In 2006 I learnt how to perform superficial TCA peels with SkinTech, and later on that year I started performing TCA medium-depth peels. During the years I have worked with several brands and products including Mene&Moy, SkinTech, Amelan, ICP, Dermaceutic, PH Formula, and Obagi. I have been fortunate enough to be able to attend seminars and some hands-on courses with several doctors known for being experts in peeling including Dr Marina Landau, Dr Jean-Luc Vigneron, Dr Philippe Deprez, and Dr Zein Obagi. I would like to thank all those experts for sharing their wealth of knowledge with me and also for their enormous efforts in writing textbooks and manuals helping us to understand skin and peels. I would like to give my special thanks to Dr Philippe Deprez for being so open and willing to share his knowledge and experience and for making medium and deep peels so accessible and easy to understand and perform.

One question I get asked very often is which peeling system is the best. Or which skincare range is the best? This is a very difficult question to answer as in my opinion all brands and products have their own place. Each range of peels or products has some fantastic and heroic life-changing products, some other great or good products, and some less-than-perfect products. I have never come across one range that has got it 100% perfect on *all* their products. Also different ranges are produced for different reasons and different needs. So it is only natural that we have to choose several product ranges to work with in clinical practice to give us all the options we need. I personally think a combination of two to four different ranges in any practice is a good choice to give the clinician the flexibility required to achieve all their goals and cater for all their patients. Let's face it: not everybody wants a deep peel, not everybody wants a superficial peel, and not everybody can afford downtime, so options are important; also with regards to products, not everybody can afford expensive products, not everybody wants a complicated skincare routine, and not everybody has the same skin colour and skin concerns. Choose around two to four skincare ranges to work with in your practice. Often these ranges will be the products that come with your chemical peels of choice, but sometimes they won't be. Choose the selection of products that will give you total flexibility when it comes to writing up skincare routines, treating skin issues, and matching your patients' budgets.

This book is not about showing you lots of before and after pictures and complicated routines. It is written with the idea to make your peeling experience easier and more practical. There are plenty of wonderful textbooks available on chemical peels, so no need to try and compete with them. My aim is rather to complement them.

Author Biography

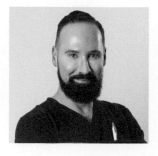

Dr Xavier G Goodarzian is the medical director of Xavier G. clinic in Southampton and London UK where he has performed chemical peels since 2006. A medical graduate of the University of Louvain (Leuven) in Belgium, he obtained member status of the Royal College of General Practitioners and has postgraduate degrees in Clinical Dermatology (Queen Mary University of London) and Cosmetic Medicine (University of Leicester) in the UK. A full member of the British College of Aesthetic Medicine (BCAM), he is an officially recognized trainer and Key Opinion Leader for SkinTech in the UK, holds training and mentoring sessions internationally, and has spoken at many live events in conferences in various countries. He is passionate about skincare, skin health, and chemical peels.

Introduction

1

WHY PEELS?

'Why peels?' you may wonder.

In my opinion there are three basic components to having a good aesthetic outcome with the majority of our patients: one is botulinum toxin, two is dermal fillers, and three is treatment of the skin itself (1).

Botulinum toxin obviously helps with smoothing dynamic lines by reducing facial expressions. It is the most popular treatment in most clinics. Repetitive use of it does improve static lines over time; however, it will not improve skin quality, nor will it target sun damage or any other skin issues.

Dermal fillers are also a wonderful tool to correct facial volume loss, to improve static wrinkles, and to improve skin hydration and skin quality over time. Of course, dermal fillers will not improve other skin issues such as sun damage or pigmentation. Skin texture does improve with repetitive use of fillers; however, it will not correct skin issues that skin care or peels may address.

So when we add skin care and peels to this heroic trio, we get amazing results as we are then fully able to address most skin issues. Chemical peels work really well in conjunction with botulinum toxin and dermal fillers.

The treatment of skin aims to reduce sun damage, reduce pigmentation, and improve skin elasticity and fine lines. There are obviously various methods for treating skin; chemical peels are one of them, but we can also mention others such as microdermabrasion, dermaplaning, microneedling, IPL, and many other types of lasers or radiofrequency and ultrasound devices available to us.

Microdermabrasion is very useful at removing superficial layers of the stratum corneum; however, I question how much indirect stimulation it provides in the deeper layers of the skin.

Dermaplaning really only removes the very surface layer of the stratum corneum, so it will have no effect on the deeper layers of the skin.

Microneedling is a good alternative to superficial peels. It helps with collagen stimulation, improvement of pigmentation, and improvement of fine lines.

Lasers, IPL, radiofrequency, and many other devices on the market all have their own place and can deliver great results; however, they all require expensive machinery, which costs a lot of money and takes a lot of space in the clinic and is generally not portable.

Chemical peels give excellent results for treating various skin issues. They are relatively quick to perform and they do not require any machinery or large capital investment of any kind. Most peels are not very complicated to learn and can yield a good level of profit for any clinic. They also allow clinicians to improve their patient's skin health by promoting a good solid skincare routine for enhancing the results and maintenance of the improvements achieved.

Peels do have their disadvantages and limitations, however. Medium and deep peels require a week of downtime, which not everyone is willing to have. Deep peels are not suitable for darker skin types, as we will explain further on. Peels like any other treatment can cause side effects, which we will discuss

DOI: 10.1201/9781003244134-1

further. Peels are also not suitable in pregnancy and breast feeding, but also some other conditions which we will discuss in further chapters.

This book will give you practical guidelines to help you grasp the basics of peeling procedures more quickly and to help you avoid complications. This book will allow you to understand peels from a much more practical point of view and will help you get going with the treatment in your clinic.

It is written for anyone who is a beginner in peelings or who has already done superficial and some medium depth peels but would like to feel more confident with medium peels and perhaps venture into the territory of deep peels.

I would still strongly recommend that you purchase a textbook about peels as well to gain more in-depth knowledge because this book is not a textbook and it is not meant to be an encyclopaedia of all knowledge about peels. We have some amazing textbooks already written on the subject. Consider this book more like a practical guide to help you incorporate peels into your practice and also to allow you to feel more confident performing them. However, be aware that this book does not in any shape or form substitute training sessions specific to each brand that you choose to use.

THE SKIN

You have all attended lectures about skin microanatomy and physiology, and for some of us it has been years since we studied it. So what do you actually remember from those lectures? Did you find them practical? Did they help you in truly understanding how the skin works? Are you able to use that knowledge and put it into practice now?

Why don't we do a quick practical recap on the skin so we get the basics right. This will be very important when it comes to understanding how peels work.

As you probably know, your skin consists of three main sections: epidermis, dermis, and subcutis or hypodermis. The subcutis or hypodermis is of vital importance for deeper skin support and fullness. It contains essential blood vessels that bring oxygen and nutrients to the skin and it has a very important role in thermoregulation. This area is generally not affected by chemical peels.

To make it easier we will now only have a look at the first two sections (2).

Epidermis (Figure 1.1) (3)

Think of the epidermis as a conveyor belt. The role of the epidermis is to create a coherent and strong barrier against the outside world, while keeping the moisture locked in. Naturally, the cells on the surface will age and die and will need to be constantly replaced, hence this constant turnover of layers upon layers of cells called 'keratinocytes'.

The lifecycle of keratinocytes starts at the bottom of the epidermis in the basal layer. The basal layer or stratum basale is a single layer of cells containing the mother cells of the keratinocytes. These basal cells sit on the basement membrane, which in itself consists of different types of collagen fibres; they give birth to new cells that get pushed upwards towards the surface. Here starts a maturation process called 'keratinization' that these cells go through till they reach the surface.

The keratinocytes are constantly changing and maturing as they move up. The first phase of this maturation process is where the cells grow extra anchoring filaments between them, called 'desmosomes'. These microscopic structures increase the strength of the bond between the cells as they mature and move upwards. These layers of cells are grouped as the stratum spinosum. So unlike the stratum basale that consists of only one single row of cells, all the other layers or strata of the epidermis consist of multiple layers of cells upon cells.

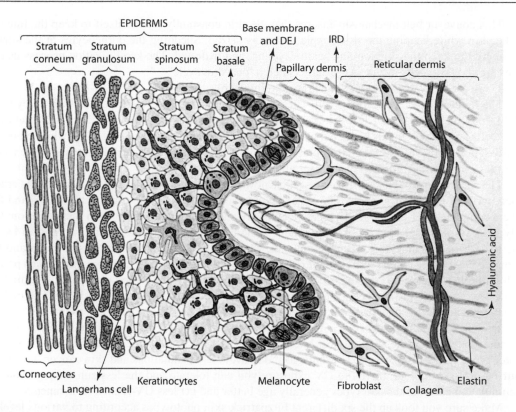

FIGURE 1.1 Microanatomy of the skin, showing normal histology. Here the epidermis and the dermis are illustrated, showing the vascular structures, the fibroblasts and the collagen and elastin fibres and pools of hyaluronic acid in the dermis. In the upper half of the illustration the epidermis is shown consisting of its many layers of keratinocytes going through the keratinization process and ending up and corneocytes at the surface. One Langerhans cell and two melanocytes with their dendritic extensions carrying melanosomes are also demonstrated.

As the cells mature, they start producing microscopic granules within them. These cells look like they have small dots or spots under the microscope, hence these layers are grouped as the stratum granulosum or the granular layer. There are two types of granules that form within these cells. One type is called the 'keratohyalin granule', which is the starting point of the creation of keratin in the cells. The other type is the lamellar body, which creates the intercellular substances that start getting secreted and fill the space between the keratinocytes.

The final stage of maturation pushes the keratinocytes into the most superficial layers where the keratin granules have filled the entire space in the cell; thus the cells have lost their nucleus and are no longer alive. These keratin-filled dead cells are flat and the space between them is filled with the substance that was secreted by the lamellar bodies earlier on. At this stage the cells are called 'corneocytes', and the many layers of these cells are grouped as the stratum corneum or the horny layer. The substance between the corneocytes consists of fatty acids, cholesterol, and other substances including the natural moisturizing factors (NMF) of the skin. Think of the stratum corneum as a wall made of bricks and mortar, where the bricks are the corneocytes and the mortar is the intercellular substance that creates an impenetrable surface.

So the stratum corneum is the most superficial part of the skin made up of dead corneocytes. The thickness of it can vary greatly according to age, body area, and how well the skin has been looked after and whether any treatments have been carried out.

This conveyor belt mechanism ensures that the skin constantly renews itself to keep the integrity of the skin while keeping the skin supple and moisturized. Shedding the corneocytes at the surface is essential to keep the skin looking healthy, young, and hydrated. The keratinization process usually takes around six weeks, which is typically called a 'one skin cycle'.

There are two other cell types worth mentioning here.

The first one is the Langerhans cell. These cells form the immune system of the skin. They play a vital role in the skin, especially when it comes to allergic reactions. We will not discuss the details of these cells any further in this book, but just think of them as mobile cells related to the white blood cell family. These cells move through the epidermis and the dermis and look for infections and agents that they may consider harmful and can trigger allergic reactions.

The second type of cell is the melanocyte. Knowledge about these cells and their activity is crucial when performing chemical peels. The melanocyte is very different to all the keratinocytes, and they have a completely different role. The melanocytes are static and do not move from their position; they only exist in the basal layer. So they sit amongst the basal layer keratinocytes in the stratum basale. The role of the melanocyte is to create melanin, which is the pigment that gives us our skin and hair colour. UV exposure increases melanin production in the melanocytes. Melanin is created via a process with multiple steps where tyrosine is converted to phaeomelanin (yellow-red pigment) and eumelanin (brown-black pigment) via an enzymatic conversion that requires the enzyme tyrosinase. The melanin is then transported in small organelles called 'melanosomes' via the dendritic extensions of the melanocytes into the keratinocytes. Once in the keratinocytes, melanin sits above the nucleus and protects the nucleus from UV radiation, almost like a mini parasol for your cells. So the role of melanin is to protect your skin from excessive UV damage and to avoid DNA mutations and skin cancer. The darker your natural skin colour, the more UV exposure you can tolerate and the less sun damage you will accumulate; hence darker skin types generally age better and get less UV-related skin cancers.

Make sure you look up the six different Fitzpatrick skin phototypes according to various levels of pigment in the skin and the reaction to UV light.

Type I: never tans, always burns, gets freckles, *usually* very fair skin with light blonde or ginger hair.
Type II: always burns, can tan a bit, *usually* fair skin and blonde hair.
Type III: can burn, can tan more easily, *usually* light skin with darker hair.
Type IV: rarely burns and tans very easily, *usually* darker skin and dark hair.
Type V: does not burn, goes very dark, *usually* very dark hair.
Type VI: does not burn, can go even darker, *usually* very dark skin and hair.

For example, I am type III. But don't be fooled as it's not as simple as that. As the stress above on 'usually' implies, your skin type is not reliably related to the way you look. My parents are both type III as well. However, I burn, then tan a bit; my dad hardly burns and tans deeper, so is somewhat like a type IV; whereas my mother cannot tan at all and in fact blisters with the slightest sun exposure, so is somewhat like a type I – and yet all three of us could be classified 'type III' because we all have light skin and dark hair.

Also many people have mixed backgrounds. So if your great grandfather was a type V and you look like you are a type III, your skin may still react like a type V; and this is exactly where the danger lies in getting side effects. So it is always important to ask about family history to ensure there is no risk of this (4).

Dermis (Figure 1.1) (5)

The dermis is the fountain of youth. Once we move below the stratum basale of the epidermis, we encounter the basement membrane and then the Grenz zone. Below this area is the start of the dermis. This entire section is called the 'dermo-epidermal junction' (DEJ) and is actually the weakest point of the skin. To reduce this weakness and to increase the contact surface between the epidermis and the dermis, these two layers do not come together in one straight line.

The DEJ consists of a coming together of what we call the epidermal invaginations and the dermal papillae. So essentially think of the base of the epidermis like fingers of a hand pointing downward while the fingers are spread out. The gaps between the fingers form the invaginations. And think of the surface of the dermis and a hand with the fingers spread out and pointing upwards. As these 'fingers' interlock, the bond between them is stronger. Now think of this in three dimensions. The entire surface of the dermis consists of these finger-like papillae coming up and matching with all the gaps of the overlaying epidermis. This is an ingenious way of increasing contact surface. The dermal papillae (the finger-like extensions) form the first part of the dermis called the 'papillary dermis'. Below this area of the dermis we enter a zone called the 'Immediate Reticular Dermis' (IRD) and then below this zone we have the reticular dermis.

The main cell of great importance to us to mention here is the fibroblast. Fibroblasts are living mobile cells that produce hyaluronic acid, collagen, and elastin fibres. So we love these cells as they keep our skin youthful and hydrated. Unfortunately, with ageing these cells become lazy and dormant and no longer readily produce these substances. The only way to increase their production in the skin is to activate them and to force them to work harder. We can achieve this by using topicals that are stimulants including retinoids and/or by performing treatments such as microneedling, chemical peeling, mesotherapy, lasers, etc.

There is a variation in the types of collagen and elastin fibres as we move through the dermis, but that's beyond the remit of this book.

REFERENCES

1. Baumann L, Saghari S, Chemical peels, in: Baumann L, ed., *Cosmetic dermatology*, second edition, McGraw-Hill, New York, 2009: 148–162.
2. Obagi ZE, Skin anatomy and physiology, in: *Obagi skin health restoration and rejuvenation*, Springer, New York, 2000: 1–14.
3. Baumann L, Saghari S, Basic science of the epidermis, in: Baumann L, ed., *Cosmetic dermatology*, second edition, McGraw-Hill, New York, 2009: 3–7.
4. Obagi ZE, Skin classification, in: *Obagi skin health restoration and rejuvenation*, Springer, New York, 2000: 65–85.
5. Baumann L, Saghari S, Basic science of the dermis, in: Baumann L, ed., *Cosmetic dermatology*, second edition, McGraw-Hill, New York, 2009: 8–13.

Classification of Peels

2

HOW NOT TO DEFINE A PEELING AGENT

Traditionally chemical peels are divided into superficial, medium, and deep peels. However, this type of classification applied to a peeling agent (or even to a percentage of a peeling agent) can be ambiguous and leaves a lot of room for individual interpretation, depending on the practitioner and the type of product or the brand they use. To make things even more difficult, manufacturers of peels often make claims about a peel being a medium peel, while in reality it is sometimes not the case. In my opinion, the most confusing peeling agent is TCA (trichloroacetic acid). TCA is often associated with medium or sometimes even deep peels, while in reality TCA can be used for superficial peels as well. So using a TCA-based peel or a peel that contains TCA amongst other ingredients does not guarantee a medium-depth peel. I think it would be best to use a more anatomical scale to determine peeling depth rather than simply relying on the peeling agent or percentage of it. Let me explain why.

Glycolic acid like most alpha-hydroxy acid (AHA) peels is used for superficial peels, usually involving the stratum corneum only; however, at high percentages with a low pH and if poorly neutralized, it can cause severe burns and involve the dermis and even lead to scarring. So glycolic acid is used for superficial peels, but it can penetrate too deep and cause damage. With most AHAs the strength of the peel depends on not only the percentage but also the pH of the acid used and also the combination of the various AHAs. It also very much depends on the time the peeling agent is left in contact with the skin and the level of neutralization afterwards.

Remember that AHAs work by loosening the bond between the keratinocytes, and this is how they can penetrate the skin by creating gaps between the cells on the surface. With TCA the mode of action is very different. TCA denatures the protein in the keratinocytes, layer by layer, and moves downward until it has run out of activity. So TCA peels generally do not require neutralization as they are self-limiting and self-neutralizing. The percentage of TCA only determines the speed of acid penetration, not the depth it can reach. So a 10% TCA could be used to obtain a very superficial peel or a true medium peel if multiple coats of the acid are applied. So again a lot of practitioners have the misconception that in order to obtain a medium peel the TCA percentage has to be at least 25%. This is not true. In fact using very high percentages of TCA such as 40% or above could be dangerous and lead to complications such as severe scarring.

Of course, it also depends on how the TCA percentage has been calculated and if the formula is stable or not. I would strongly recommend that you buy reputable brands of TCA peels that have been created with safety in mind. Please do not buy neat TCA or just water-based TCA and use it on a patient. Always follow the manufacturer's guidelines.

Always remember that the depth of penetration of any peel is greatly affected by the type of products used for skin preparation. For example, the use of retinoids prior to a peel will increase the depth of any peel, so please bear this in mind.

DOI: 10.1201/9781003244134-2

HOW TO DEFINE A PEELING AGENT ON A MORE ANATOMICAL SCALE

From an anatomical point of view a very superficial peel would involve the stratum corneum. With TCA superficial peels, the stratum basale or even the Grenz zone could be involved. Peels involving the papillary dermis above the immediate reticular dermis (IRD) are considered medium peels. The agents used here are usually TCA or phenol or a combination of both. Any peels involving deeper layers below the IRD are considered deep peels and the safest agent to use for this type of peel is phenol (Figure 2.1).

I would like to draw your attention to two different types of classification compared to the traditional method. I find Philippe Deprez's model (Figure 2.2) very useful.

The Wiest and Schürer model (Figure 2.3) is also interesting and gives further clarification to the traditional method (1). Comparing this classification with the Deprez model, we can see that the upper epidermis would correspond to level 1, the middle and deep epidermis would correspond to levels 2 and 3, the upper papillary dermis would correspond to levels 4 and 5, the papillary dermis would correspond to level 5, and the mid-reticular dermis would correspond to level 6. This is a far better classification than the traditional 3 level approach; however, I feel that the Deprez classification gives a more accurate view of the actual level of peeling.

We will see in further chapters what the effect of penetrating these different levels is and also how that will have a direct effect on the downtime.

Now you may think, why do we actually need various peeling depths? If a superficial peel is safer to perform, should we not just stick to using them? Or if a deep peel has a longer downtime, why do we actually need to perform them?

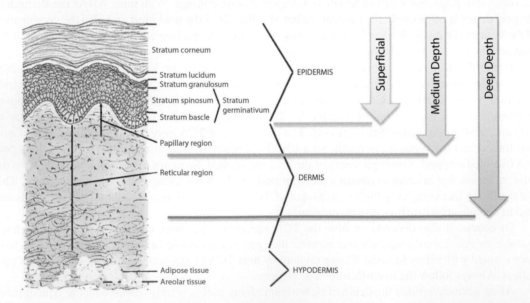

FIGURE 2.1 Traditional peeling depths in a cross-section of the skin with its histological features. The three main layers of the skin are highlighted. Superficial peels only involve the epidermis, medium peels involve the papillary dermis above the IRD, and deep peels involve the reticular dermis below the IRD. (Courtesy of SkinTech Pharma Group.)

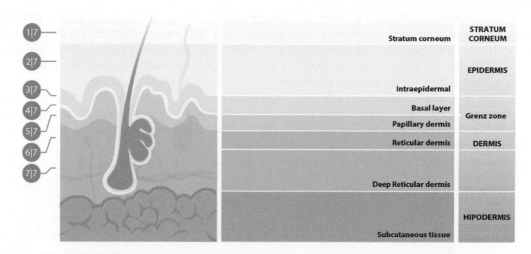

FIGURE 2.2 Dr Deprez's peeling scale of seven penetration depths, illustrated with a cross-section of the skin showing the three main layers of the skin. The skin is further divided into seven layers: stratum corneum is a level 1 peel; intra-epidermal peels are level 2; basal layer peels are level 3; the Grenz zone is level 4; a peel to the papillary dermis is level 5; reticular dermis is level 6; and finally a deep reticular dermis peel would be a level 7. (Courtesy of SkinTech Pharma Group.)

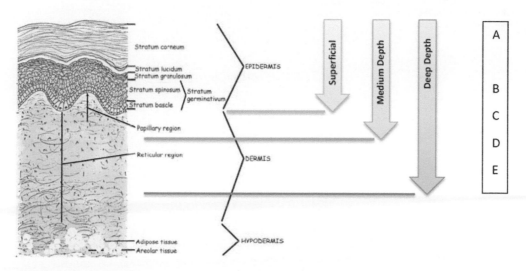

FIGURE 2.3 Wiest and Schürer skin depth classification, showing the ABCDE method of indicating skin peeling depths: A, upper epidermis; B, middle and deep epidermis; C, upper papillary dermis; D, papillary dermis; E, mid-reticular dermis.

The peel that we choose has to have a logical reason behind it. If the aim is to freshen up the skin and create a glowing surface, a superficial AHA peel would be very suitable. If we wanted to remove more sun damage or pigmentation, a superficial TCA could work. However, with most superficial peels a course of peeling sessions is required. So the patient will need to commit to a course of four to six sessions to get the desired result.

With a medium-depth peel a lot more sun damage could be removed in one session and pigmentation or even acne scarring could improve more dramatically; however, compared to a superficial peel that has little to no downtime, a medium-depth peel will have a downtime of roughly five to ten days, depending on the skin and the preparation before the peel. So it is more effective and there is more collagen and elastin formation, but longer downtime.

A deep peel is only indicated if wrinkles are to be removed or if a more intense enhancement of skin elasticity is required. This type of peel is extremely effective in removing wrinkles and tightening the skin; however, it requires at least a week of social isolation and further downtime until the skin settles down properly.

I will explain more about these different peeling types in further chapters.

REFERENCE

1. Deprez P, Peeling classification, in: *Textbook of chemical peels*, second edition, CRC Press, Boca Raton, 2016: 1–6.

Consultation
How and When to Recommend Peels

3

THE CONSULTATION

The consultation process for peels is not so different from a normal medical consultation except for a more in-depth talk about the patient's skincare routine. It is possible that your patient has booked the consultation to ask about chemical peels, in which case you can be prepared to ask the relevant questions. It is also possible that your patient has come in with a specific concern and is asking you to offer a solution, in which case you need to evaluate whether a peel would be suitable to improve the problem. Some patients may not have considered a peel before the consultation as an option, while some may have but are not sure or have been put off by looking at pictures online and are worried about pain and downtime.

Concerns that may be improved with a chemical peel are:

- Fine lines and wrinkles
- Loss of skin elasticity
- Sun damage
- Lentigines
- Uneven pigmentation
- Melisma
- Post-inflammatory hyperpigmentation (PIH)
- Active acne
- PIH caused by acne
- Acne scarring
- Stretch marks

To start the consultation, first of all listen carefully to the concerns of the patient. Ask them what brings them to you. See how they describe their problem and how it affects them physically and mentally. Ask open questions to begin with and also find out if they have looked into possible treatments or if they have considered peels before as a solution.

Once the initial introduction has finished, start asking more specific questions.

Past cosmetic history: which treatments have they received in the past? You should try and find out all the treatments that they have had on their face so far – not just those related to the current

DOI: 10.1201/9781003244134-3

concern but also in general. Then ask more specifically about any treatments that have been done so far for the current concern – any previous peels? Microdermabrasion? Topical products?

It is important we find out about previous treatments because it allows us to ensure that it does not potentially cause issues with a peel but also to make sure that they have not already had the treatment that we had in mind previously.

Medication: ask patients to list all the drugs that they are currently taking, including any topical creams. This is very important because some drugs can make us more UV-sensitive or can increase skin permeability. This could potentially cause side effects if it causes the peel to penetrate too deep. A good example of this would be isotretinoin oral medication for acne; patients should be off this drug for at least six months before a chemical peel can be carried out as it increases skin fragility and could cause scarring. Another example is tretinoin cream and also benzoyl peroxide cream; both topicals increase skin permeability and could cause the peel to go too deep.

Unfortunately most patients do not think about their creams when they list their medication, so it is important that we actively ask about those.

Allergies: remember to ask about any allergies to any oral medication, any antibiotics, and any topicals.

Family history: if in any doubt about skin typing, then ask about family history. As explained previously, some people have a mixed background and their skin may react to peels with issues relating to a darker skin type than their own actual skin type. So for example a person who has skin type III may have Caribbean ancestors and therefore may have issues that a skin type V may encounter after a peel.

Medical history: make sure you take a full and thorough medical history, like any other medical procedure. Previous illness? Chronic illness? Hereditary illnesses? Auto-immune illnesses? Psychiatric history?

Expectations: make sure you find out what they expect from the treatment and make sure that their expectations are realistic. You will need to explain all the requirements for a peel, the skin preparation and importance of aftercare, and how to cope with the downtime. Also it is really important to explain that a superficial peel will not give the same result as a deep peel, which is what most people think a superficial peel does!

TALKING ABOUT PEELS

Often I get asked by colleagues how I talk to my patients about peels and how I 'convince them' to have a peel, especially medium or deep peels with longer downtimes. The answer is I don't ever convince anyone to have any procedure done. I simply assess the problem during the consultation and find out if a peel could be one of the solutions; I then offer the peel as an option. It is important, however, to explain why a peel would be a good idea. Some patients are happy to have a peel after one consultation. For some others it may take a while before they come round to the idea, and they may opt for other options in the meantime.

Let's look at two examples:

A patient comes in with lentigines as a concern. You know that they have developed these lentigines due to excessive sun exposure over the years, even though they may swear that they have never been in the sun (which always makes me laugh, by the way). Treatment options could be:

- Simply use good topicals including skin-lightening agents and sun protection.
- Have cryotherapy on the individual lentigines.
- Have a course of fraxional laser sessions.

- Have a course of superficial TCA peels.
- Have one or two medium-depth peels.

Then explain each option and the potential outcome and downtime. Of course, you can explain which option would give them the best result in your opinion, but ultimately they have to choose depending on what is acceptable to them in terms of downtime and budget.

Another example is peri-oral lines. Treatment options could be:

- Anti-ageing topicals such as tretinoin cream
- Mesotherapy
- Microneedling
- Dermal fillers and or botulinum toxin
- A course of fraxional laser treatments
- A few medium-depth peels
- A one-off deep peel

Again, explain each option and explain the possible outcome with each option with the necessary downtime and cost (1).

PATIENT CONCERNS ABOUT PEELS

The word 'peel' sometimes scares the patients, so in that case it is important to talk them through the downtime and recovery process. For some patients it may take several exposures before they opt for a peel, so if you really believe a deep peel is the best option for someone, keep mentioning it every time you see them and you will find that soon patients become interested and start asking more questions, which eventually leads to them having the treatment, with great results.

The two specific points that most scare patients about peels are pain during the procedure and downtime. It is, however, important to mention that non-chemical peel options may also be as painful (if not more) and may have the same – or a more severe – downtime than a peel! So it's important to differentiate the aspects of different peel depths and explain what is relevant for the type of peel you are talking to them about.

Let's see what points we should discuss for various peels during the consultation process.

- Superficial peels
  - Can improve very fine lines, skin elasticity, sun damage, pigmentation, acne, rosacea, skin hydration, etc.
  - Procedure is not painful, just some tingling which only lasts a maximum of five minutes.
  - There is very little downtime, just some minor peeling and dryness for a couple of days.
  - Usually a course of four to six peels is required to achieve optimal results.
- Medium peels
  - Can improve fine lines and wrinkles, skin elasticity, sun damage, pigmentation, acne, and acne scarring.
  - Procedure is moderately painful for about ten minutes but analgesia will be given to help.
  - Downtime is visible peeling for five to seven days.
  - Usually one or two peels are enough to give good results.

- Deep peels
  - Can remove lines and wrinkles and sun damage and give a remarkable improvement in skin elasticity.
  - The pain level really depends on if only a local deep peel is applied or the full face is treated. For localized deep peels, the pain is similar to a medium peel and analgesia will help.
  - Downtime is seven to ten days with a minimum seven days of isolation.
  - One peel usually gives excellent results.

PROTOCOLS

For the majority of people, a full-face deep peel is an option they have never considered before. So during the first consultation various options should be discussed as above. Once a patient has decided that a full-face deep peel is what they wish to go ahead with, I will always do a second consultation to go through the process in depth, and I will ask them to bring their partner or next of kin with them to ensure that all their questions have been answered. Even if they have looked into deep peels already and come specifically to talk about it, a second consultation with their partner or next of kin is strongly advised.

Once I have explained the entire process of prepping, peeling, downtime, and aftercare, I show the patient and their partner multiple pictures of patients at various levels of healing so they can visibly see what the patient will look like. This is really helpful as it stops them both from panicking and not knowing what is normal after such a peel. At that stage the before pictures are taken, the peel date is set, the medical forms are given to the patient to take home, read, and complete, and the necessary medication is prescribed for the patient.

First Consultation

Some patients come to me specifically for a full-face deep peel, because they have been recommended or referred by my medical colleagues or they have been referred by their friends or relatives who have already had a deep peel with me. These are the best type of patients because they are generally very motivated and well-informed to some degree. They do not mind travelling from the other side of the UK to come and see me and don't mind spending a couple of nights locally just a one-minute walk down the road from my clinic in a very comfortable hotel.

Some patients come to me for other reasons, and the first thing that comes into my mind is 'I would love to give you a phenol peel' when I see the usual sun-damaged skin with severe laxity and solar elastosis. Obviously, however, that's not the way to approach these patients. They may have come to me for something totally not related to their skin – perhaps they have come for botulinum toxin treatment or want bigger lips or are concerned about a mole on their face. For these patients it may take a while before the subject of skin health is discussed. Always remember that most people genuinely believe that their skin is in a much better state than it actually is. So to tell someone who has never considered their skin as an issue that they need a full-face deep peel would almost be an insult. Over time these patients may actually discuss the subject with you or ask about options to improve their skin and then a deep peel could be offered as an option. Or they may see some leaflets or booklets or before and after pictures in your clinic or on your website and that might inspire them to ask.

Some patients come into a consultation to ask about improvement of their skin or sun damage. This is an easy one, of course. For anyone who has deep lines and wrinkles and solar elastosis, I am confident that a phenol peel would give them amazing long-lasting results, and I am very happy to discuss it and offer it as a solution. At this stage I do not go into detail about it. I do, however, show them some before and after pictures and also pictures about a real patient's recovery journey.

I give them enough information and leaflets so they can go and do their own research and think about it. I also ask them to come for a second consultation with me so we can go through the procedure in more detail. I always ask them to bring a significant other with them for this second appointment – ideally, the same person who will be with them for the first 48 hours after the procedure.

Second Consultation

During the second consultation I assess the face again and explain the procedure in detail. I specifically go through all the preparation steps and explain exactly what will happen during the peel itself. I also am very detailed about the aftercare and what needs to happen in the first ten days after the peel. I also show a lot of pictures of the procedure and also how they might look immediately after the peel and for the first ten days after. I insist that this is in the presence of the spouse or next of kin or carer who will be with them during the first few days of the recovery.

I make sure that all their questions have been answered. I do not lie about the commitment it takes to have this peel, and I do make sure they understand that the first four to eight hours after the peel will be relatively painful, but manageable with analgesia.

A thorough medical history is taken, and the consent form is explained. I usually send the patient home with the consent form to read carefully in their own time and sign and bring back as the deep peel consent form is too long to read in the clinic.

Patient Preparation

Before pictures need to be taken from all angles. Make sure that the before and after pictures are always taken in the same place in your clinic with the same lighting. This will ensure good comparable before and after pictures.

Take pictures from the front view, three-quarter view, and side profile on both sides. Make sure the hair does not cover any part of the face.

What I also always recommend to patients is to have botulinum toxin treatment one or two weeks before their peel procedure. This allows the new skin to heal without excessive muscle movement, which ultimately gives a much better result and improves dynamic and static lines. This is definitely very important for deep phenol peels, as you will read further on; however, it would also be preferable before superficial or medium peels.

During the consultation we obviously talk about skincare. As mentioned before, the prep and aftercare products should be an integral part of the peel. How do we talk about these products, and how do we get our patients to use them and stay compliant?

There are two preliminary principles. First of all, no cream, no peel. If a patient is not willing to take or use the products, I will not offer them a peel. It's very simple. Second, I don't want them simply to continue using their usual products as that means I have no control over what is being put on the skin.

For patients who have no skincare routine at all, I explain the importance of a twice-daily routine and the importance of sun protection. This is actually the easiest group to deal with; however, make sure that your routine is simple to follow and does not involve more than three steps twice daily.

For patients who already use products or have a routine (which is the majority of our patients), I explain the importance of the appropriate skin prep products. On a rare occasion I may allow them to use one or two of their own usual products and incorporate them into the routine I give them, if I know the product very well and if I know for certain that it will help improve skin prep and will not cause any side effects. Otherwise, I will ask them to put all their products to the side and only use the peel preparation products and sun protection as instructed.

For patients who are product junkies and have a million products and think they know everything, I will ask them to bring their products with them at the next session so I can have a look and see if any of their products may be good to use after the peeling process is over. So this way I can help to simplify their routine and get rid of unnecessary products, but ultimately they have to stick to my skincare routine for prep and aftercare.

I always write down the recommended skincare routine step by step (with steps in the morning and steps at night). Then I keep a copy of this information in the patient file so I can refer back to it. This step is crucial to help the patient stay compliant with the routine. If you do not write this down for the patient, I can guarantee that they will make mistakes and either omit a step or use them in the wrong order or even use day products at night and vice versa. I have even had patients not washing off a cleanser and putting cream on top of an unwashed cleanser. So please do not assume that people know how to use products. If a cleanser needs to be washed off, write it down in brackets after the cleansing step. Also write down the amount of product to be used for each product – a pea size? Half a fingertip? A full fingertip? And to which area of the face do they apply the product – the entire face? Only on the areas of concern?

The clearer you are with your instructions, the more likely it is that they will stick to this. This step of explaining and writing down the skincare routine can, of course, be delegated to an assistant or therapist who has been trained by yourself, who you can trust to do the job as well as you would do. Be specific with when you want the patient to start the skin prep step: a minimum of two weeks is required, and for some procedures in some skin types, it may be six weeks or even longer.

REFERENCE

1. Deprez P, Selection of the right peel, in: *Textbook of chemical peels*, second edition, CRC Press, Boca Raton, 2016: 32–44.

Patient Journey

Steps Leading to and from the Peel

4

After the consultation a treatment plan is set up to allow the patient to prepare for their peel treatment(s) and the aftercare stages after the treatment.

STAGES FOR EACH TREATMENT TYPE

Superficial Peels

Since superficial peels have the least downtime, prep time could be as little as two weeks. Before pictures should be taken and then the patient should be given their prep products to take home and start the prep process.

On the day of the peel, an aftercare or after-peel product will be applied to the face. It is best for the patient to go home immediately after any peel and not spend too much time outdoors.

During the desquamation phase the patient should use the aftercare products given by the clinician.

Depending on the peel type or the peel system used, superficial peels are repeated every one to four weeks. So after the desquamation period, the patient should go back to using the prep products to get ready for the next peel.

The desquamation with superficial peels depends on the agent used. With an AHA (for example, Neostrata glycolic peel) or BHA (for example, Obagi blue peel radiance) typically some skin dryness and very minor skin flaking is visible. With a retinol peel (for example, Neostrata Retinol peel) the dryness and flaking are a bit more obvious. With a superficial TCA (for example, SkinTech Easy TCA) the skin flakes are larger. Most superficial peels recover after three to five days.

Medium Peels

For a medium peel the prep time could be as little as two weeks if the patient is of skin phototype I or II. Even with phototype III, I would recommend a longer prep period (for example, SkinTech Unideep or

DOI: 10.1201/9781003244134-4

Easy TCA Pain Control). With phototypes IV, V, and VI, prep time should be at least six weeks, which is considered to be one skin epidermal cycle. Some medium-depth peels require even two to three skin cycles of prep before a medium peel is considered safe. A good example of this is the Obagi Blue peel (1).

After the peel and aftercare product is applied to the face, it is strongly recommended that the patient just goes home to rest after the treatment. Typically during the first two days after a medium TCA peel some oedema may be present, which can be most noticeable in the peri-orbital and peri-oral regions.

The patient should have relative rest for the period of five to seven days that follow to allow appropriate healing of the skin. Exercise is not recommended during this time due to sweating. For the first couple of days after a medium TCA peel there is no flaking; however, the surface of the skin feels like a layer of plastic and feels very tight. It is important to avoid excessive facial movement during this time to avoid premature detachment of the skin.

Washing hair and a long soak of the face under the shower is not allowed in the first few days. From day three onwards the area around the mouth may already start cracking and peeling. The flaking will really become noticeable on days four to five and will most likely end by days seven to ten. The better the skin prep has been, the quicker the skin will heal and recover.

It's really important for the patient to stick to the aftercare instructions given. Pulling the skin off or scratching may lead to scarring or infection. Only the recommended aftercare products should be used. After the skin has peeled, it is still recommended to continue with the aftercare products for at least another two to three days. The skin will be sensitive, so going immediately back to the prep products on day seven may cause some irritation.

Medium peels can be repeated if required; however, a period of four to six weeks is recommended to allow the skin to settle before the next peel.

Deep Peels

Since deep peels are not performed on phototypes IV, V, or VI (although some practitioners have been known to treat type IV), the prep time for this peel type can be as little as two weeks. However, due to the fact that this is a seriously invasive procedure, most patients do book this sometime in advance, which allows for a longer prep time anyway.

Once the second consultation is done and the patient is happy to go ahead with this peel, the before pictures should be taken, and the patient will be given the prep products to start using at home. A week or two before the peel, full-face botulinum toxin treatment should be performed to avoid an exacerbation of dynamic lines after the peel. At the same time any other investigations can be carried out, which will be explained in a further chapter.

Any prescriptions for medication will be written at the same time, ready for the peel.

After a phenol peel, the area of the peel is covered in a yellow powder consisting of bismuthsubgalate (BSG), unless an occlusive tape is applied first for 24 hours (this will be discussed later). It is imperative that this powder is not removed or washed off under any circumstances for seven days. So washing of the hair or the face is not allowed during this time.

Patients go immediately home after such a peel and must rest completely for at least three days. We will discuss the details of deep peels later.

After the yellow crust has come off on day eight, the skin can be washed and it will be very erythematous and sensitive. So it is important that only the aftercare creams given by the clinician are used and nothing else.

CONSENTING AND AFTERCARE

Patients need to be consented to any type of peel. The consent form has to explain the procedure and explain potential undesirable outcomes. Make sure your consent forms are thorough, especially for deep peels, including contra-indications (2).

There follow some examples of the information to appear on consent forms and aftercare sheets.

Consent for Treatment with a Superficial Medical Skin Peel (AHA, BHA, Retinol)

Preparing the Skin for a Superficial Peel

For chemical peels to be successful and to reduce possible side effects, you will have to use specific creams given to you by your practitioner for at least two weeks before the actual procedure.

These creams are not meant to make you feel better or smell nice. Some of these are medicated, pharmaceutical strength products that are as important as the peeling procedure itself. They might make your skin dry and red and cause some peeling. This is intended to happen and is a sign of activation of your skin.

There will also be specific skincare advice after the peel which will enhance and maintain the result of your peel. Again, it is very important to use them appropriately and not to risk using any over-the-counter products which could potentially cause allergies and side effects.

Please remember that **the sun (or actually any visible daylight)** contains a lot of UV radiation and is the primary cause of ageing of the skin. This ageing process starts as early as the age of 30 when collagen production drastically slows down. Any chemical peeling is meant to reduce and possibly reverse some signs of this ageing. The deeper the peel, the more improvement can be expected.

However, the face should **not be exposed to sun (or daylight) without full UV protection**. Failure in taking this measure could potentially end up causing side effects such as sunburns and pigmentation on the face and of course would reduce the efficacy of the peel you have just invested in.

You should never go outdoors at any time of the year without UV protection and should never actively try to tan your face. Remember tanning is not safe and always indicates damage to the skin with alterations to the DNA structure of your skin cells and ultimately loss of elasticity, breaking down of collagen, wrinkles, pigmentation, and in some cases, skin cancer including malignant melanoma, which can be deadly. Using sunbeds is completely out of the question.

If you have any questions or concerns regarding your skincare, please contact us for advice, but do not deviate from your plan in any way unless advised by your practitioner.

About the Superficial Peel Procedure

Medical skin peels with acids are used to treat ageing skin and photo-ageing of the skin, to improve problems of abnormal pigmentation caused by the sun, and to give the skin a younger, fresher appearance.

They are also very effective in the treatment of active acne and can arrest even severe cases of acne for 6–12 months, often eliminating the need to take drugs.

Medical peels are **not** beauty treatments; they are medical procedures with the potential for adverse side effects.

A solution of acid is applied to the face (neck, decolletage, and hands may also be treated) by your practitioner. This will sting or tingle for a few minutes but is tolerable, and most patients do not require any anaesthesia or analgesia.

The peel is then finished by the application of a post-peel cream or the acid being washed off, depending on the type of peel you are having. You may then need to take home a prescribed cream to apply to the treated area for the next few days (as directed).

Immediately following the peel, the treated skin may look red, and for a few hours to 24 hours the treated skin looks smooth and quite tight.

Depending on the type of peel chosen and discussed with you, the peel may need to be repeated. For superficial peels this will usually be a course of four to six peels, each spaced about two to four weeks apart.

Who Should Not Have a Chemical Peel?

- If you have a history of problems with **keloid scars** (raised scars that grow out beyond the original site of injury) or other types of scarring of your skin;
- If you have facial warts or any current facial infection;
- If you have used the anti-acne treatment **isotretinoin** (brand name Roaccutane) within the last 12 months;
- If you have darkly pigmented skin. In such cases, you would generally be unsuitable for the deeper peels owing to the potential for skin bleaching. Afro-Caribbean or Asian skin is often not suited to facial peels because of the risk of bleaching the skin. This is particularly the case with the deeper peels where the top layers of skin are removed. Your practitioner will discuss this.

Summary of Risks from Medical Skin Peels

Peels are a commonly used form of skin rejuvenation and the vast majority are carried out with no complications. Adverse effects from skin peel are extremely rare. However, you do need to be aware of the risks, which can be summarized below:

- Burning sensation and stinging.
- Redness – can last for a few days.
- Peeling – it is important that you do not pick at or peel off the skin.
- Sensitive skin after the peel.
- In rare cases, patients may experience an infection in the skin or an outbreak of cold sores. This normally only occurs in patients who have a history of such complaints and anti-viral medication may be recommended if such complications occur.

- Mild transient swelling of the face.
- Hypo- or hyperpigmentation – patients must use all aftercare products as directed and remember to use a high-factor sunscreen (factor 30 or more).
- In rare cases scarring or keloids may occur.

Patient Declaration and Agreement

A medical skin peel treatment for skin ageing, photo-ageing, over-pigmentation, and active acne has been explained to me by my practitioner.

I also understand and accept the following:

I understand and accept each point below:	Patient Initials
• Loose skin must not be pulled or picked off; otherwise there could be a risk of scarring.	
• Cold sores (herpes simplex) around the mouth can be triggered off by the peel in those who have previously suffered from cold sores. I understand I must therefore tell my practitioner before the peel if I have *ever* suffered from cold sores so that preventative tablets can be prescribed.	
• I understand that the aftercare instructions advised by my practitioner must be *strictly* followed. In particular, strict sun avoidance and the use of a high factor (30+) UVA and UVB block when outdoors must be complied with for at least three months to minimize any risk of over-pigmented areas developing, triggered by the sun. This also relates to cloudy and dull days when the sun is not visible.	
• I understand that the results of treatment with a skin peel cannot be guaranteed, and I consent to undergo treatment having been fully informed of the benefits and possible risks of treatment.	
• I accept that the use, indications, risks, and benefits of the peel have been explained to me by my practitioner.	
• I confirm that I have had the opportunity to have all my questions answered to my satisfaction, including clarification of any words or phrases used that I am unsure about.	
• I understand that the practice of medicine (like surgery) is *not* an exact science and therefore that no guarantee can be given as to the results of the treatment referred to in this document.	
• I accept and understand that the goal of this treatment is improvement, not perfection, and that there is no guarantee that the anticipated results will be achieved.	
• I also accept that it may be necessary to have **further** peel treatments to achieve the result that I desire and that each additional treatment or adjustment will be charged for.	

The treatment, the risks and benefits, the side effects, and the expected outcomes have ALL been explained to me. I have read and understand the information I have been given in this entire document, and I consent to undergo this treatment entirely at my own risk.

Patient's name (print): _____

Patient's address (print):   _____

_____

Patient's Signature: _____   Date: _____

Practitioner's Signature: _____   Date: _____

Aftercare Sheet for Superficial Peels

WHAT SHOULD YOU DO AFTER A SUPERFICIAL PEEL PROCEDURE?

It is very important that you carefully follow the advice given by your practitioner following a peel treatment to help improve the benefit of the procedure and reduce the risk of complications or side effects. This includes:

- Using all the creams as directed and using a high-factor sun protection cream every day.
- Cleansing the face gently with a soap-free cleanser, patting dry with a towel, and moisturizing twice a day.
- Not picking off any dead/peeling skin as this may cause bleeding and/or discoloration, or even mild scarring.
- Not exposing yourself to the sun without sunscreen for at least six weeks after treatment to reduce the risk of hyperpigmentation (brown blotches on the face). A high-factor sunblock should be used daily to protect the skin (even on a dull or cloudy day).
- If itching is severe during the healing phase, antihistamines may be recommended to help stop this.
- Avoiding scratching at the skin to reduce the chances of scarring.
- Contacting your practitioner immediately if you notice any signs of infection, scarring, or pigment changes.

Consent for Treatment with a TCA Skin Peel (Superficial or Medium)

Preparing the Skin for a TCA Peel

Preparation is the key to success! You can't just decide to have a TCA chemical peel. You have to allow time for your skin to be **prepared** with skincare. For any chemical peel to be successful and to reduce possible side effects, you will have to use specific creams given to you by your practitioner for at least four weeks before the actual procedure.

These creams are not meant to make you feel better or smell nice. They are **not cosmetics** that can be purchased over the counter. They are medicated, pharmaceutical-strength products that are as important as the peeling procedure itself. **They might make your skin dry and red and cause some peeling. This is intended to happen and is a sign of activation of your skin.**

There will also be specific skincare advice after the peel which will enhance and maintain the result of your peel. Again, it is very important to use them appropriately and not to risk using any over-the-counter products which could potentially cause allergies and side effects.

Please remember that **the sun (or actually any visible daylight)** contains a lot of UV radiation and is the primary cause of ageing of the skin. This ageing process starts as early as the age of 30 when collagen production drastically slows down. Any chemical peeling is meant to reduce and possibly reverse some signs of this ageing. The deeper the peel, the more improvement can be expected.

However, the face should **not be exposed to sun (or daylight) without full UV protection**. Failure in taking this measure could potentially end up causing side effects such as sunburns and pigmentation on the face and, of course, would reduce the efficacy of the peel you have just invested in.

You should never go outdoors at any time of the year without UV protection and should never actively try to tan your face. Remember: tanning is not safe and always indicates damage to the skin with alterations to the DNA structure of your skin cells and ultimately loss of elasticity, breaking down of collagen, wrinkles, pigmentation, and in some cases, skin cancer including malignant melanoma, which can be deadly. Using sunbeds is completely out of the question.

If you have any questions or concerns regarding your skincare please contact us for advice, but do not deviate from your plan in any way unless advised by your practitioner.

About the TCA Peel Procedure

Medical skin peels with TCA acid are used to treat ageing skin, photo-ageing of the skin, improve problems of abnormal pigmentation caused by the sun, and give the skin a younger, fresher appearance. They are also very effective in the treatment of active acne and can arrest even severe cases of acne for 6–12 months, often eliminating the need to take drugs. TCA peels are not beauty treatments; they are medical procedures with the potential for adverse side effects.

A solution of trichloroacetic acid (TCA) is applied to the face (neck, decolletage, and hands may also be treated) by your medical practitioner. This will sting for a few minutes but is tolerable, and most patients do not require any anaesthesia. In some cases, with some medium peels, analgesia may be prescribed for you to take 30–45 minutes before your peel.

A fan is used to relieve any stinging and further layers are applied until the correct depth of penetration is achieved, as judged by the experience of the medical practitioner. The peel is then finished by the application of a post-peel cream, and the patient takes home a prescribed cream to apply to the treated area for the next few to seven days (as directed).

Immediately following the peel, the treated skin may look red and for the next 24–48 hours the treated skin looks smooth and quite tight. It is not uncommon for the face or treated areas to swell for a day or so.

The skin then becomes tighter, drier, and sometimes darker as any abnormal pigmentation comes to the surface. On about the third day, the skin will start to peel and this is similar to the peeling sometimes seen after sunburn. The post-peel cream can be liberally applied and the skin must be allowed to peel naturally without any pulling-off of loose skin. On the fifth to seventh day, the peeling is complete and the skin looks fresher and smoother.

Depending on the peel you choose, your face (or treated area) may be significantly peeling for five to ten days, so you may experience social pressure or wish to remain indoors during this time, away from normal social and work activities.

Depending on the type of TCA peel chosen and discussed with you, the peel may need to be repeated. For lighter (superficial) TCA peels this will usually be a course of three to four peels spaced about two weeks apart. For deeper (medium or deep medium) TCA peels you may need only one peel, but another may be required after about six weeks.

The final results can be seen and assessed over a period of four to six months after the (final) peel, not before. During this time the skin will produce more collagen and will become younger in structure, tighter, and more elastic.

What Should You Do after a Peel Procedure?

It is very important that you carefully follow the advice given by your practitioner following a peel treatment to help to improve the benefit of the procedure and reduce the risk of complications or side effects. This includes:

- Using all the creams as directed and using a high factor sun protection cream every day.
- Cleansing the face gently with a soap-free cleanser, patting dry with a towel, and moisturizing twice a day.
- Not picking off any dead/peeling skin, as this may cause bleeding and/or discoloration, or even mild scarring.
- Not exposing yourself to the sun without sunscreen for at least six weeks after treatment to reduce the risk of hyperpigmentation (brown blotches on the face). A high-factor sunblock should be used daily to protect the skin (even on a dull or cloudy day).
- If itching is severe during the healing phase, antihistamines may be recommended to help stop this.
- Avoiding scratching or picking at the skin to reduce the chances of scarring.
- Contacting your practitioner immediately if you notice any signs of infection, scarring, or pigment changes.

Who Should Not Have a Chemical Peel?

- If you have a history of problems with keloid scars (raised scars that grow out beyond the original site of injury) or other types of scarring of your skin.
- If you have facial warts or any current facial infection.
- If you have used the anti-acne treatment isotretinoin (brand name Roaccutane) within the last 12 months.

- If you have darkly pigmented skin. In such cases, you would generally be unsuitable for the deeper peels owing to the potential for skin bleaching. Afro-Caribbean or Asian skin is often not suited to facial peels because of the risk of bleaching the skin. This is particularly the case with the deeper peels where the top layers of skin are removed. This will all be discussed with you, and appropriate pre-peel products may be given to you to avoid pigmentary complications.

Summary of Risks from Medical Skin Peels

Peels are a commonly used form of skin rejuvenation, and the vast majority are carried out with no complications. Adverse effects from TCA skin peel are extremely rare. However, you do need to be aware of the risks, which can be summarized below:

- Burning sensation and stinging.
- Redness – can last for a few weeks.
- Peeling – it is important that you do not pick at or peel off the skin.
- Sensitive skin after the peel.
- In rare cases, patients may experience an infection in the skin or an outbreak of cold sores. This normally only occurs in patients who have a history of such complaints, and anti-viral medication may be recommended if such complications occur.
- Mild transient swelling of the face.
- Hypo- or hyperpigmentation – patients must use all aftercare products as directed, and remember to use a high-factor sunscreen (factor 30 or more).
- In rare cases scarring or keloids may occur.

Patient Declaration and Agreement

A TCA medical skin peel treatment for skin ageing, photoageing, over-pigmentation, and active acne has been explained to me by my practitioner.

The treatment is administered by applying a mask solution on to my skin. This stings somewhat but is relieved by a fan. The mask is then taken off and a post-peel cream is then applied. Immediately afterwards the treated skin will look red (like sunburn) and this redness will fade over a day or so.

The next day the skin will feel tight and may still have a slight redness. Later that day, or the next, it will become drier and tighter. The post-peel cream must be applied as directed by my practitioner. The skin may also become darker as any areas of over-pigmentation dry and come to the surface.

On day three or four day the skin will start to peel (like the peeling after sunburn).

The peeling must be allowed to occur naturally and no loose areas of skin should be pulled off or there could be a risk of scarring.

The post-peel cream should be applied as directed. After seven to ten days the peeling should be completed.

I also understand and accept the following:

I understand and accept each point below:	Patient Initials
• Loose skin must not be pulled or picked off; otherwise, there could be a risk of scarring.	
• Cold sores (herpes simplex) around the mouth can be triggered off by the peel in those who have previously suffered from cold sores. I understand I must therefore tell my practitioner before the peel if I have *ever* suffered from cold sores so that preventative tablets can be prescribed.	
• I understand that the aftercare instructions advised by my practitioner must be *strictly* followed. In particular, strict sun avoidance and the use of a high factor (30+) UVA and UVB block when outdoors must be complied with for at least three months to minimize any risk of over-pigmented areas developing, triggered by the sun. This also relates to cloudy and dull days when the sun is not visible.	
• I understand that the results of treatment with TCA skin peel cannot be guaranteed, and I consent to undergo treatment having been fully informed of the benefits and possible risks of treatment.	
• I accept that the use, indications, risks, and benefits of the TCA peel have been explained to me by my practitioner.	
• I confirm that I have had the opportunity to have all my questions answered to my satisfaction including clarification of any words or phrases used that I am unsure about.	
• I understand that the practice of medicine (like surgery) is *not* an exact science and therefore that no guarantee can be given as to the results of the treatment referred to in this document.	
• I accept and understand that the goal of this treatment is improvement, not perfection, and that there is no guarantee that the anticipated results will be achieved.	
• I also accept that it may be necessary to need *further* TCA peel treatments to achieve the result that I desire and that each additional treatment or adjustment will be charged for.	

The treatment, the risks and benefits, side effects, and expected outcomes have ALL been explained to me. I have read and understand the information I have been given in this entire document, and I consent to undergo this treatment entirely at my own risk.

Patient's name (print): _____

Patient's address (print): _____

_____

Patient's Signature: _____ Date: _____

Practitioner's Signature: _____ Date: _____

Aftercare Sheet for a Medium Depth Chemical Peel

Post-peel Instructions for You to Read and Follow:

Please note that your face will **feel very tight** for the next **five to seven days** and that **some swelling**, especially in the region of the eyelids is normal. As you have read on the consent form you signed before the treatment, you must **NOT** pick off any of the skin areas when flaking. If, however, you have areas of loose skin, you may use scissors to cut them off, but you must not pull the skin off by force at any time.

It is also normal for your skin to develop a darkish brown colour before it comes off. The new skin growing underneath will be pink for up to a week after the peeling has finished.

It is best to avoid washing your hair for the next three to four days, and when you do, please remember not to let soapy water run down your face.

Please do not wash your face today (the day of the peel). The doctor has applied an ointment on your face (skin recovery cream) which should stay in place until tomorrow morning (the day after the peel). From tomorrow (the day after the peel), you may wash your face very gently with just lukewarm water or a very small amount of gentle liquid cleanser.

Please **do** reapply the skin recovery cream **immediately after** washing (apply the cream a minimum of twice a day, but it can be more if necessary). You should **not** use any other creams or products on your face whilst your skin is peeling.

Please do not use any of the products you were given to prepare your skin with **before** the peel until you have seen the doctor two weeks after your peel; at that point he or she will advise you what skincare routine to go on.

Whilst peeling it is extremely important to avoid infections.

Please avoid close contact with pets and small children.

Whenever you touch your face, you must wash your hands with soap thoroughly beforehand.

The healing process should be pain-free. If you have any painful or tender areas, you must ring the clinic.

Also if you notice any signs of cold sores coming up, contact us immediately.

CONSENT FOR TREATMENT WITH A PHENOL (DEEP) PEEL

Introduction

Phenol (carbolic acid) **peels** are the strongest kind of chemical skin peels available and are generally used on severely aged skin characterized by deep wrinkles and significant skin laxity. The procedure is a serious medical treatment and should not be entered into lightly and without a lot of thought and preparation.

In principle, the results of a phenol peel are permanent, but of course after the peel the skin will continue to age, bringing about normal skin changes due to ageing. Sensible care and protection of your skin will, however, help to perpetuate the benefits of the peel. Results are not immediate, and it will take a few months to judge the final result.

As explained during your consultation, this procedure usually consists of a deep peeling of the whole face or parts of the face, including the upper and lower eyelids and the skin around the lips, where most of us suffer from prominent lines and wrinkles.

Your visit to the clinic for the actual peel will take around two to four hours. This includes the peel itself and also time for you to relax after the procedure so that we are able to observe you for a time before you are able to go home.

You will need to be accompanied by a 'Supporting Person' (next of kin or friend/relative) for the procedure, and they must be able to take you home and stay with you for at least 48 hours. You will *not* be able to undergo the procedure without this Supporting Person.

The role of your Supporting Person is very important and you should choose this person carefully because they will have important responsibilities to fulfil both before and after your peel.

It is extremely important that you understand not only what the procedure involves and what you need to do in order to be prepared for the procedure but also how **you** can help to avoid developing unwanted side effects or complications.

This Patient Information Pack contains a detailed explanation of the procedure itself and the steps necessary. Please take your time to read it, not just once, but a few times in order to **fully** understand it and help you formulate any questions you may have for your practitioner before you agree to undergo the procedure.

We also strongly recommend that your Supporting Person reads this document so that they can understand what you will be going through and what they will need to do to help you.

GENERAL SUN (UV) DAMAGE ADVICE – WHY OUR SKIN AGES PREMATURELY

The sun (or actually any visible daylight) contains ultraviolet (UV) radiation. This is the primary cause of ageing of the skin. Any chemical peeling procedure is designed to reduce and possibly reverse some of this skin ageing. The deeper the peel, the more improvement can generally be expected.

For good facial skin health, the face should never be exposed to sun (or daylight) without full UV protection, at any time of the year. Even on cloudy days, one should not go outdoors without some form of UV protection, and one should not actively try to tan the face.

Remember 'tanning' **cannot be** and **is not** safe and **always** indicates **damage** to the skin, with alterations to the DNA structure of your skin cells taking place. Over time, this ultimately leads to a loss of elasticity due to a breaking-down of collagen and elastin fibres (the skin's natural 'scaffolding' support structures), wrinkles, pigmentation, and possibly skin cancer, including malignant melanoma, which can be fatal.

Using sunbeds to achieve a tan is completely against sensible medical advice because it delivers damaging UV radiation to your skin and simply accelerates the above process.

The condition of and damage to your skin **today** is a result of **years** (often decades) of UV exposure (whether daily unprotected general exposure, tanning in the sun, or from sunbeds). This is what we are seeking to improve by carrying out this peel procedure.

In addition, other factors such as smoking and poor nutrition can affect the health and condition of your skin. It is of course sensible – for so many reasons – NOT to smoke, and if you are a smoker undergoing this peel procedure, now is perhaps a good time to stop.

THIS PEEL IS A SERIOUS *MEDICAL* PROCEDURE AND NOT A 'BEAUTY' PROCEDURE

Please remember that this peel is not a 'quick-fix' beauty procedure. It is a serious medical and invasive procedure, and you are embarking on a 'Treatment Journey' that will take time.

Your Treatment Journey involves having consultations, visits to the clinic, and blood tests before the peel. The procedure itself is very technical and involves a lot of preparation by **you** the patient, and the doctor.

During the process of determining your suitability for a phenol peel you will be required to complete a medical history questionnaire. You must ensure that you complete it fully and disclose any and all relevant information about your past and current medical status – including providing a full list of any medication you are taking.

There is also a list of contra-indications (reasons why one should not have this peel), which is included in the medical history so that we can ensure that you are suitable for the procedure.

AFTER YOUR PEEL

It is important to note that after your peel, you must adhere to strict sun avoidance and skin protection. Failure to do so could result in unwanted side effects such as severe sunburns and abnormal pigmentation on the face, and of course it would reduce the effectiveness of the peel you have just invested in.

Immediately after the peel, parts of or indeed your whole face may be covered in bandages (depending on the procedure carried out – according to your 'problem areas').

You will probably not be able to open your eyes due to swelling of the face (often, the whole face), including the eyelids shortly after your peel, and this will possibly last for up to 48 hours.

On the day of your peel (day zero), your 'Supporting Person' will be required to take you home after the procedure, but only after you have been observed by staff in the clinic for a while, to ensure your fitness and health to leave the clinic.

Your 'Supporting Person' will be required to stay with you for at least 48 hours to assist you at home with basic needs, supporting help, and for your safety. They will also need to bring you back to the clinic the **day after** your peel (day one).

You will be advised about appropriate medication to take home to relieve any pain.

Once the bandages are removed from your face the **day after** the peel (day one), we will cover your face with a yellow powder which will then 'set' like a mask/crust for seven to eight days.

Once you return home with this powder applied, you will **not** be able to leave your home (or place of recovery) for that period of time.

You will not be allowed any solid foods from the time you have the peel until the crust-like mask has been removed on day seven to eight.

You should also refrain from excessive movement of the face – especially the mouth area – in order to promote even healing of the skin. Therefore, you will not be able to open your mouth too widely or brush your teeth as you would normally do. Using a straw to drink liquid food and using mouthwash only to clean your teeth is strongly recommended.

Botulinum Toxin treatment may have to be performed one or two weeks before the peel to help relax active facial muscles in order to promote even healing of the skin. This will be discussed with you.

You will of course not be able to smoke during this time! This is *very* important and you must commit to this. This is perhaps a good opportunity to give up smoking.

You will also need to return to the clinic on day three **and** day six for a checkup to ensure the healing process is progressing to the doctor's satisfaction. You **must** attend these appointments.

On day seven or day eight, the mask can be removed by yourself at home; then you will be reviewed at the clinic the next day to look at the interim results and healing. Your face **will** be red/pink for perhaps another week or longer. This redness is normal and will settle down over the following weeks. You can, of course, use makeup to cover this.

Your skin will continue to improve over the next couple of months. After three months you should see the full effect of the peel. The slight swelling that you experienced after the peel should have settled, and new collagen fibres will have formed in your skin, which should provide a tightening and lifting effect on the whole face.

YOU MUST HAVE REALISTIC EXPECTATIONS OF THIS PROCEDURE

Please bear in mind that **not all lines and wrinkles** can always be removed. The key message is 'improvement but **not** perfection'.

Remember, the condition of and damage to your skin **today** is as a result of **years** (often decades) of UV exposure, so you must be realistic about what may be achieved.

Some areas of deep wrinkling or deep acne scarring might need an additional touch-up with the same peel within the first month after the peel. This can be discussed with the doctor and may be chargeable.

NON-SERIOUS SIDE EFFECTS

It is possible to develop milia (a 'pearly' white lump of dried sebum – the skin's natural oil) during the healing phase. This is a **normal** reaction, and these milia can be simply extracted with a very small needle in the clinic.

It is also possible to develop telangiectasia (very small thread veins on the face) during this time. This will generally settle down on its own, but occasionally might need some treatment (such as laser) after the healing is complete. If this is needed, this will be an additional chargeable treatment.

You must avoid heavy lifting, pushing or pulling heavy weights, straining, or any exercise during the initial healing phase to avoid over-production of these thread veins. Hence, taking some laxatives for example in the first couple of weeks is recommended to prevent straining while passing on the toilet.

PREPARATION BEFORE YOUR PEEL IS KEY TO SUCCESS

You cannot 'just decide' to have this chemical peel when you wish. You must allow time for your skin to be prepared with appropriate skincare and the day of the actual peel is determined around a strict number of visits to the clinic before and after the peel – all of which you must attend.

For any chemical peel to be successful and also to reduce possible unwanted side effects or complications you will have to use specific skincare provided to you for at least two weeks before the actual procedure.

There will also be specific skincare creams for you to use **after** the peel, which will enhance and maintain the result of your peel. Again, it is very important to use them as directed.

Do not risk using **any** over-the-counter shop-bought skincare products at the same time as this could potentially cause allergies, reactions, and unwanted side effects.

MEDICATION

You will have to take some antibiotics and/or antiviral medication before the peel and during the healing phase to avoid infections such as bacterial infections or a flare-up of herpes simplex (cold sores). These will be provided for you.

YOUR PHENOL PEEL 'TREATMENT JOURNEY'

Step-by-step instructions for your peel, in day order

Step 1

Your Consultation and Information Gathering

The consultation with the doctor is the first and very important step in preparing yourself for the peel.

You will be given information about the treatment and its risks and benefits to you, and you will be examined/assessed to ensure that the procedure is deemed appropriate for you.

You are given this Patient Information Pack to take away with you to study it carefully at home, in your own time.

You should take all the time **you need** in order to consider all the implications of undergoing this procedure. This includes the effects on your personal life, social life, and work.

You should also think about the psychological/emotional pressures you will be faced with during the first week or two. Remember all the implications explained in this document, such as: you will be unable to eat solid food for the first week; you **cannot** smoke; you will need a Supporting Person to help you; you will have a 'mask' on your face for about a week; you will be 'stuck indoors' for a week, so will need things to keep you occupied, etc. **These all have to be considered by you and indeed your Supporting Person.**

Please also take the time to discuss this treatment with your next of kin/partner (and Supporting Person if different). Let them read this Patient Information Pack.

You do need both physical and emotional support to be able to undergo this treatment.

Once you have decided that you wish to proceed with the peel, you will need to book the next stage of your Treatment Journey – Step 2.

Step 2

'Before' Photographs, Consent Form, Start the Pre-peel Skincare, Investigations, and Fees

During this visit we will take detailed photographs of your face. These photographs will be your 'before pictures'.

The visit is also an opportunity for you to ask further questions to help in deciding to proceed. You will be asked to sign the Consent Form.

The pre-peel skincare starter pack will be given to you, and you will be shown how to use each item – see section on skincare.

We will arrange necessary investigations as required – such as blood tests and possibly an ECG after taking a detailed medical history – and you will be asked to complete and sign a medical history questionnaire.

It is VERY important that you complete this medical history questionnaire fully and truthfully. Even if you think an aspect of your **current** health or **past** health is not important, you must still disclose it and we will decide whether it will have an effect on your suitability to undergo the peel.

This visit will also give you the opportunity to discuss payment options for the whole procedure.

Step 3

Finalize Paperwork, Revise Investigations, and Examine Your Skin (One Week Pre-peel)

We will now review all the paperwork and look at all your test results.

We will also look at the state of your skin and possibly adjust the skincare plan if necessary to have the skin as ready as possible for the peel.

Step 4 (Peel Day Zero)

The Day of Your Phenol Peel

You must arrive one hour prior to the peel. You must **not** smoke!

Do Not Eat Any Food Two Hours before the Peel

You will be given some medication and will sit and relax for a while before your peel.

During the Procedure

You will be fully conscious during the procedure, and don't worry if you are nervous.

Your blood pressure and oxygen in the blood will be monitored at all times.

Your face will be cleansed and disinfected.

You might receive some intravenous fluids.

Your face will finally be numbed with some local anaesthetic injections into the skin, and the peeling solution will then be carefully applied to the face.

Immediately after the Peel

You will be given some analgesia (pain relief), and your face **may** be (partially) covered in a mask that must stay in place until the next day when you will need to return to the clinic for Step 5. Note: If a mask is not applied, then you do not need Step 5, but you will be told by the doctor if this is the case.

It is extremely important that this mask stays in place overnight; otherwise the peeling process will not occur evenly and it will adversely affect the outcome.

Avoid any facial or mouth movements.

Drink plenty of fluids and liquid food through a straw. You must stay hydrated.

Please refer to your post-peel information leaflet for further details.

Step 5 (Day One Post-peel)

Removal of Bandages and Application of Mask Powder

At the clinic, the mask (if one was applied) will be taken off the day after the peel.

Your face will be cleaned, and it will then be covered by a regenerative powder which will 'set' like a firm crust over your face.

If no mask was applied on the day of your peel, this powder would have been applied to your face immediately after the peel so there would be no need to attend the clinic for Step 5.

Step 6 (Day Three Post-peel)

Your First Checkup

On day three after your peel you will be checked to ensure that your skin is healing without any problems and that there are no signs of any infections or other side effects.

Some areas of the face may be 'touched up' with some Vaseline or Fucidine ointment.

You **must** attend this appointment.

Step 7 (Day Six Post-peel)

Second Checkup

On day six you will be checked to ensure that your skin is healing without any problems and that there are no signs of any infections or other side effects.

More areas of the face may be 'touched up' with some Vaseline or Fucidine ointment.

Step 8 (Days Seven to Eight Post-peel)

Removal of Mask Powder

On days seven to eight you will be required to remove the crust-like powder mask at home by yourself after applying more and more Vaseline or Bepanthen ointment to the face.

THE DAY AFTER REMOVING THE MASK you will attend the clinic to see how your skin has healed.

How you remove the mask at home will be explained to you, and it is contained in the post-peel information leaflet.

Step 9 (One Month after Peel)

First Follow-up for Progress Review and Photographs

During this visit, the quality of your skin will be assessed, and some photographs might be taken.

A skincare plan will be discussed again with you to ensure further improvement and skin recovery.

A possible peel touch-up in certain areas can be discussed at this stage if necessary.

Step 10 (Three Months after Peel)

Second Follow-up for Progress Review and Pictures

During this visit we will take some 'after pictures' because by month three you should be able to see the lifting effect of the peel and your skin should look and feel appreciably improved.

Step 11 (Six Months after Peel)

Third Follow-up for Progress Review and Final Pictures

This will be your final visit to the clinic as part of the peel journey.

Your final 'after pictures' will be taken at this stage, and it is now that we can assess the effectiveness of the peel procedure – not before.

Checklist of things to remember after peel and until day eight

- Do not smoke!
- Have access to mouthwash because using a toothbrush is not allowed for eight days.
- Have cotton buds available to use to clean your eye corners.
- Have straws available to drink your liquids and liquid-based food.
- Wear comfortable nightwear with an open front so you do not disturb your face when putting it on or taking it off. The same with clothes.
- Plan for eight days of liquid or semi-liquid food.
- You will be unable to wash your hair for eight days.
- Do not use hair dye for at least two days **prior** to the peel and three weeks **after** the peel.

Possible complications and side effects

There is a relation between depth of the peelings and level of risk; it must be borne in mind that a deep peeling involves a much higher risk of complication than a superficial one.

- Itching of the face.
- Redness of the skin for at least ten weeks.
- Appearance of thread veins and/or milia on the face.
- Pigmentation abnormalities: areas of light or dark skin.
- Abnormal healing.
- Scarring.
- Insufficient results.
- Transitory or definite change of skin colour depending on peeling.
- Infections.
- Ectropion or entropion of the eyelids (inversion or eversion of the eyelid).
- Acne type reaction.
- Demarcation line (neck to jawline).
- Dilated pores.
- Benign re-pigmentation of moles.
- In the case of complete face deep phenol peelings, the general toxicity of the phenol acid should be considered. However, prior blood analysis is required and we monitor your progress and body functions during the procedure – including cardiological examination.
- Anaphylaxis (severe allergic reaction).

Contraindications (who should NOT have this peel):

- Patients who are pregnant or breast-feeding
- Patients with history of keloid or hypertrophic scarring
- Patients with severe auto-immune illnesses
- Patients with skin collagen diseases (for example, Ehlers Danlos syndrome)
- Patients with skin infections
- Patients with active cold sores
- Patients with dark skin types, unless appropriate peel is chosen and anti-tyrosinase products are used
- Patients with cancers under treatment including radiotherapy
- Patients who have had recent surgery such as face-lifts in the last six months
- Patients who have taken oral Isotretinoin (Roaccutane) in the last 12 months
- Patients who use IMAO antidepressants
- Patients who have Insulin-dependent diabetes
- Patients with heart disease and arrhythmia
- Patients with kidney disease
- Patients with liver disease
- Patients with severe respiratory illnesses
- Patients with severe anxiety and or claustrophobia
- Patients with a low pain threshold
- Patients who are used to taking a lot of analgesia of any kind

I confirm that, to the best of my knowledge, none of the above contra-indications apply to me.

Patient Signature _____ Date _____

Aftercare Sheet for a Phenol Peel

Please also refer to your initial Patient Information and Consent Pack for full in-detail explanation about the procedure and all your necessary appointments at the clinic.

Please also refer to your list of medication as explained day by day.

After resting for a while in the clinic, you will be able to go home, accompanied by your nominated Supporting Person who should remain with you and attend to your needs for 48 hours.

Immediately after the Treatment

You may feel a burning or warm sensation to your face for a few hours. This is easy to control using the pain-killers that are provided to you.

If you have taken antivirals or antibiotics, continue to take them as instructed.

Start **drinking fluids** again as soon as possible. Food must be liquid or semi-liquid for several days in order to avoid chewing movements which will cause excessive facial movement.

About eight hours after the peel it is normal for a liquid-type substance to 'flow' or collect beneath the adhesive mask. This liquid is *lymph fluid* and is normal – it will be dried-up when you return to the clinic the next day by applying a yellow regenerative powder after removing the adhesive mask.

In areas not covered by the adhesive bandage, oedema (swelling) and redness will occur for the first 24–48 hours. **Under no circumstance remove the adhesive tapes yourself!**

It is possible that you will not be able to open your eyelids completely for two days, or at least the first morning after the peel. This effect will be more significant the looser the eyelid skin was before the peel. **This reaction is normal, it is a sign that the treatment has worked well.** Within a maximum usually of 48 hours you will be able to open your eyes properly, read, watch television, and occupy yourself as you see fit.

You should remain in a comfortable armchair or lay down, but with your head higher than your heart in order to facilitate a reduction in the swelling. It is best to remain somewhere quiet with subdued lighting, perhaps listening to music. Avoid talking, laughing, grimacing, smoking, or moving the face in any way. **The skin needs to remain still to repair itself properly.**

Accompanied by your Supporting Person, you must return to the clinic to have the adhesive mask removed (if this was applied) and have a yellow regenerative powder mask applied 24 hours after the peel. If you had any areas not covered by the adhesive mask after the peel, they would have already been covered by a yellow regenerative powder mask immediately after the peel.

CHANGING THE MASK (*24 hours after the peel*) = **day one** (*Step 5*)

After 24 hours, you return to the clinic to have the first adhesive mask removed if this was applied.

Any residual impurities will be removed from the skin and it will be 'retouched' if necessary.

The second mask, consisting of the yellow regenerating powder, will be applied. As explained above, if no adhesive mask tape was applied to the skin, this yellow powder would have already been applied after the peel. **This yellow powder forms a crust when applied and must stay on your skin for the next six to seven days.**

UNDER NO CIRCUMSTANCES SHOULD YOU TRY TO REMOVE THIS CRUST FROM YOUR FACE UNTIL DAY SIX TO SEVEN WHEN IT IS READY TO COME OFF. FAILURE TO FOLLOW THIS INSTRUCTION MAY RESULT IN INFECTION AND SEVERE SCARRING OF THE FACE!

FROM DAY ONE TO DAY SEVEN

On the day the adhesive mask is removed and the following day you must apply the yellow regenerative powder we give you if necessary in order to complete this yellow regenerating mask.

You will need to apply more yellow powder if the mask becomes green, because this means it has become a bit wet. **You should reapply a bit of yellow powder to keep this mask dry and yellow.**

Note: The area very close to the eyelids must not be covered in yellow powder. Simply apply FUCIDINE ointment whenever the skin starts to crack and hurt a little.

A 'cardboard-looking' mask will thus develop from the yellow powder. This mask is made up of the regenerating powder only and does not contain skin particles.

If you accidentally get some powder in your eyes, do not panic; just clean with a cotton bud and administer a drop of ARTIFICIAL TEAR.

As explained in your Patient Information and Consent Pack, **on DAY THREE** (*Step 3*) you will return to the clinic for a short checkup by the doctor, followed by another visit on **DAY SIX** (*Step 7*) before you remove the yellow mask yourself on **DAY SEVEN OR EIGHT.**

IT IS ALSO ADVISABLE TO REFRAIN FROM SMOKING TO AVOID PUCKERING THE LIPS, AVOID GETTING TOO HOT TO PREVENT SWEATING, AND MOVE THE FACE AS LITTLE AS POSSIBLE.

EXERCISE IS STRICTLY NOT ALLOWED FOR AT LEAST THE NEXT TEN DAYS!

Continue to take the prescribed medication.

From DAY FIVE onwards pieces of the mask may start to come off. **Do not pull them off.** Instead apply a bit of Vaseline ointment to the deepest cracks in the powder mask to keep the area moist and clean.

During the evening of **DAY SEVEN** (i.e. Tuesday evening if your peel was carried out on the previous Tuesday), apply a thick layer of Bepanthen or Vaseline to your face before going to bed.

ON DAY EIGHT (e.g. the Wednesday if you had the peel on a Tuesday the week before)

You should reapply the Bepanthen ointment in the morning. Apply this ointment to the remaining parts of the powder mask with your hand four to six times during that day. Each time, leave the cream in place 10–15 minutes, then rinse your face in warm (not hot) water and wipe it gently with your fingers or a cloth. If the powder seems very hard, you can soften the mask by 'kneading' it so it slides off easily.

There is no risk involved here as the skin has already repaired itself. The mask you are trying to remove is made up of skin debris, which is not attached to your new skin, and if the mask does seem to cling to the face, it is because of the hairs on your face.

Parts of this mask might have already started to come off from DAY SIX. Hard pieces may, however, remain stuck around your eyes in the areas in which there was no powder mask. If they do not slide off, apply a thick layer of Fucidine ointment and wait. This area sometimes takes longer to heal.

DAY NINE = *the day after the mask removal*

You will generally have an appointment at the clinic for a checkup. However, the checkup may be postponed, in which case you will have a telephone conversation with the doctor.

Normally, the whole mask will have come off by now. If this is not the case, reapply the Bepanthen ointment.

The skin will look pinkish, smooth, and radiant. There may still be some slight inflammation. If you wish, the makeup you chose before the peel can be applied to hide the redness.

The full effect of the peel is best observed six months after the procedure, so do not try to judge the result until then.

You will be reviewed in the clinic at **months one** (*Step 9*), **three** (*Step 10*), **and six** (*Step 11*) after your peel for checkups and photographs. At month six we will be able to present you with a copy of your before and after photographs if you wish.

REFERENCES

1. Obagi ZE, Skin health: The concepts, in: *Obagi skin health restoration and rejuvenation*, Springer, New York, 2000: 27–46.
2. Deprez P, Phenol: Contraindications, precautions and safety, in: *Textbook of chemical peels*, second edition, CRC Press, Boca Raton, 2016: 264–268.

Skin Prep

5

Let's talk about skincare. Appropriate skin preparation before a peel allows the peel to penetrate easier and more evenly, and because the skin is already in good condition and in an active state, it allows for better and faster healing. By using specific products, specific concerns can also be improved, such as pigmentation or acne, and specific side effects can be reduced, such as post-inflammatory hyperpigmentation (PIH) (1,2).

What do I mean by skin being in an active state? As we age our skin becomes lazier and the epidermal turnover slows down, which means we have an accumulation of corneocytes at the surface, thus a thickening of the upper epidermis. These dead cells make the skin look dry, dehydrated, and dull. They also accumulate a lot of sun damage and excess pigment. So the more superficial layers of the skin are all dead cells, which makes it harder for active ingredients to penetrate appropriately; also because the turnover is slow, the healing and replacement of those layers will be more difficult after peeling. Ageing also has a dramatic effect on the dermis. The fibroblasts have far less activity and produce much less collagen, elastin, and hyaluronic acid. This results in skin dryness, thinning of the dermis, and the appearance of wrinkles and skin laxity.

By using a good skincare routine with specific active ingredients, we can change this or we can at least start the process so the peel has a better effect and the skin can recover more quickly. This process of making the skin more active does not happen overnight and requires weeks of preparation. One epidermal cycle is around six weeks. In an ideal world everyone should prepare their skin for at least six weeks to go through one cycle and get healthier cells throughout the skin before the first peel. This is not necessary for superficial and some medium peels, but six weeks or more prep time would still give the best results. It should be noted this is very much peel-dependent, and it is always best to follow the instructions from each manufacturer to get optimum results.

The effect of skin prep on the epidermis is sometimes called epidermal compaction. This means that the majority of the dead corneocytes have been removed and the epidermis mostly consists of healthy living and well-functioning keratinocytes. Longer prep time will also even create an activation of the fibroblasts, which leads to much faster healing and an improved collagen and elastin production.

AN IDEAL SKINCARE ROUTINE

So what is an ideal skincare routine?

- Twice daily
- Not too complicated
- Not too many steps
- Logical order of products
- Logical reason for the use of each product

DOI: 10.1201/9781003244134-5

The face has to be cleansed twice daily (morning and night). As a rule of thumb, thinner, more liquid products such as gels and serums are applied first before lotions or creams. Sunscreen should be the last step in the morning before the application of makeup. Some people have told me over the years that they apply a moisturizer over their sunscreen. This is totally wrong and it just proves the lack of understanding of the logic behind skincare in some people.

Cleansers

Is 'cleanser' not just a fancy name for soap? No! Cleansers have an acidic PH, like the skin itself. Soaps are generally alkaline.

It is best to use cleansers that are rinsed off with water rather than milky lotion-based cleansers as they provide a better cleansing action. Rinse-off cleansers can be very gentle too, so even sensitive skin types should be able to use them. For oilier skin types this is essential.

One word of caution is to ensure that we do not over-cleanse the skin, especially with harsh products as this will damage the skin's lipid barrier and cause irritation. Some people with oily skin get obsessed with cleansing and I know some who wash their face with harsh products three to four times daily to remove any oil residue. Long term this is damaging and should be avoided. So generally a twice daily cleansing routine should suffice.

It is best to remove any makeup with wipes or a cleansing milk first before cleansing. Cleansing is about cleaning the skin, not about just removing makeup. Sometimes it is actually best to do a double cleanse, which means cleanse and rinse off once and repeat again to get the best cleansing action. This can be done in the shower or at the sink. Wet the face first with lukewarm water and apply a pump of your cleanser to the palm of your hand and make it foam in your hands, then massage thoroughly onto the entire face and then rinse off with water.

Toners

Cleanse, tone, moisturize is the good old adage from many years ago. Why do we need to use toners? Is it really necessary? Unlike most popular belief, toners are not designed to remove cleanser residue from the face and they are not meant to shrink your pores. Also toners should ideally be alcohol-free to avoid damaging the skin's natural lipid barrier. Toners have got an acidic PH so by lowering the PH after cleansing, they improve the penetration of further products being applied. But I have to be honest, if someone is on a tight budget or wants a simple routine, the toner would be the first product I would remove from the routine.

Some toners come in a handy spray form, so they can simply be sprayed onto the face with a fine mist. Some toners come in the form of pre-soaked pads. These are very handy too as they are very practical. Most toners, however, just come in a bottle and one needs a cotton pad to apply them.

Toners often also contain active ingredients, such as vitamins, anti-oxidants, AHAs, BHAs, and sometimes even retinoids. So in this case they do a lot more than just lowering the PH. They actually have a very active role in the skincare routine. Sometimes different toners with different active ingredients can be used for day and night. This is obviously very brand-specific.

Once the toner has been applied, wait a minute or two for it to dry before going onto the next step.

Gels

Gels are very light products that hardly leave any residue on the skin. These are ideal agents to use for application of medication on to the skin, such as benzoyl-peroxide, metronidazole, retinoic acid (although cream versions of retinoic acid are much more popular), and many other topical antibiotics.

Gels would typically be applied before any other product (but after the toner). They can be used once or twice a day according to the frequency required by the individual product.

Serums

Serums are light products that could be completely or partially transparent. Generally they contain concentrated active ingredients such as vitamin C, vitamin A, vitamin E, bakuchiol, retinol, AHAs, and so on. Serums are generally used twice daily, although some are more specific for day use and some specifically for night use. Serums are the ideal vehicle to deliver a lot of active ingredients onto cleansed and toned skin, as the skin is ready to receive all the active ingredients after the first two steps.

Serums should be applied after the application of a gel (especially if medicated). Different serums may also be layered on top of each other if necessary for their specific active ingredients.

Creams

Do we need to moisturize? The simple answer is, no, we don't have to, unless absolutely necessary to avoid excessive skin dryness. Moisturizers themselves are not anti-ageing products, especially if they have no anti-ageing ingredients in them. The majority of moisturizers on the market, including the very expensive ones endorsed by many celebrities are just a mixture of oil, water, emulsifiers, stabilizing agents, and perfume. So apart from creating a film of mineral oil on the skin, they have no other purpose. They make your skin appear more hydrated as the oil film on the surface gives you that false sense of security, but in fact there is no benefit to the skin.

A moisturizer should ideally be completely devoid of mineral oil and should have active ingredients that provide an anti-ageing effect. Most medical-grade products have many wonderful moisturizers with specific ingredients to achieve certain results. So rather than using a moisturizer, I would prefer to use a serum and follow with a sunscreen. If you suffer from skin dryness, by all means choose a moisturizer, but at least get one with the active ingredients that your skin needs.

When performing chemical peels, there is of course a time and place for moisturizers and repair creams to allow the skin to recover. This is very important for the healing period after a chemical peel. For superficial peels this could just be a few days. For medium peels this could be ten days or more, and for deep peels this could be as long as six weeks or more. It is very important to have these recovery creams or repair moisturizers as part of the skincare package for the patient. After a peel the skin is simply too sensitive to immediately go back to active products with, for example, AHAs or retinoids. This of course needs to be explained during the consultation, during the peel procedure, and again after the peel procedure to ensure patients know what to do with their products at home.

Do we need day and night creams?

The simple answer is it depends. Day creams tend to have a lighter texture and some contain some SPF as well. Night creams are richer in texture and may contain ingredients that destabilize in sunlight. However, there are many creams that are designed to be used both in the morning or at nighttime. In general, day creams should be about protection and night creams should be about repair.

Again to make the routine simple for the patients and also to keep the cost at an acceptable level, it is often preferred to use a cream that could be used twice a day.

Sunscreen (3)

Do we need to use a sunscreen daily? Yes absolutely. Every single day! No matter what the weather is like. The majority of the damage to the skin is caused by UV light. So it is extremely important that we educate our patients in the importance of sun protection, not just while undergoing (a course of) chemical peels, but also generally on a daily basis. The sun's UVB and UVA rays are both very damaging, but UVA has a more deeply penetrating effect; remember that UVA passes through clouds and glass, so windows will not protect you from UVA. Most sunscreens are broad spectrum, which means they do protect against UVB (the SPF value) and against UVA (the star or plus-sign rating).

Sunscreens are divided into chemical (such as octocrylene) and physical (such as zinc oxide) screens. It is recommended that zinc oxide always be present in a good quality sunscreen as it gives one of the best spectrum protections.

There are many sunscreens available nowadays that are specific for the face and are very cosmetically acceptable, meaning they are completely translucent after application and they are not oily and just feel like a very light moisturizer. I would personally recommend a factor 30 or more on a daily basis.

How much sunscreen should we use on the face? I would say at least a fingertip to ensure full coverage of the entire face.

Remember to apply all your creams including the sunscreen with the tip of your fingers and not the palm of your hands unless you want to waste half of the product being applied on the palms of your hands.

Makeup

Can I apply makeup over my sunscreen? Yes, of course. I would personally recommend mineral-based makeup to avoid oily products on the skin but also to avoid putting unnecessary chemicals onto the face.

My pet hate is: 'my makeup contains SPF so I don't need a sunscreen'. You do! Makeup will not give you enough sun protection on its own, unless it is a specific makeup with high SPF designed to be used as makeup and sunscreen in one.

Figure 5.1 shows an example of application of decent amount of a good broad-spectrum sunscreen to the left cheek. Even though to the naked eye there is not much to see, under the Observ filter we can see the effect of UV protection in that area.

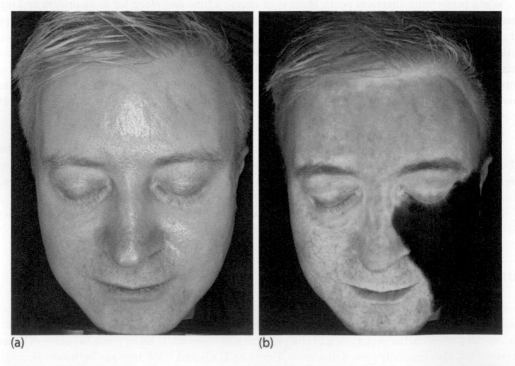

(a)   (b)

FIGURE 5.1 (a) Broad spectrum sunscreen is not visible when applied to the left cheek, but the difference in UV protection is seen in (b) under the Observ filter.

INGREDIENTS

Let's now look at some ingredients in products.

For a full list of ingredients and a full explanation of how each of these works, please refer to any text book. What follows is just a quick list of the most popular ingredients in products with a simple, easy-to-understand explanation that you could use to explain to your patients.

Anti-Oxidants (4,5)

Anti-oxidants are amazing substances that neutralize free radicals caused by UV radiation. They have a huge anti-ageing benefit. They are best used in the morning but can also be used at night as well. Vitamin C or ascorbic acid is the one that is most commonly used in various skin serums. Ferulic acid and resveratrol are also quite popular. So the combination of an anti-oxidant rich serum and a sunscreen is the perfect duo for a great morning anti-ageing routine.

Most anti-oxidants come in the form of serums. This allows great penetration of the product into clean and prepared skin.

Alpha-Hydroxy-Acids (6)

Alpha-hydroxy acids (AHAs) are very popular in serums and creams because they help exfoliate the dead layers of corneocytes, reduce pigmentation, and improve skin hydration. They improve skin texture and are perfect for thinning out the top layers of the epidermis to allow better penetration of other active ingredients and peels. As you will know, there are various AHAs available and often a combination of them is used. They all have roughly the same function but some have slightly more specific additional functions as well. Examples of AHAs are glycolic acid (penetrates fastest and deepest and exfoliates), lactic acid (slightly larger molecule so slower penetration, thus more gentle), mandelic acid (better effect on acne), azelaic acid (effective for acne but also pigmentation), phytic and kojic acid (good for pigmentation), and so on.

AHAs can of course be combined with anti-oxidants and other active ingredients to give the best results.

Beta-Hydroxy-Acids

The only beta-hydroxy-acid (BHA) used in products is salicylic acid. It has a larger molecule and is lipophilic compared to the hydrophilic AHAs, so it penetrates best through the hair follicle and is great for oily and acne-prone skin. Often AHA-BHA combinations are used in products or peels.

Retinoic Acid (7–9)

There is so much written and studied about retinoic acid. There is plenty of evidence that it is an excellent anti-ageing product. Retinoids are a group of substances that have an effect on the skin at the cellular level. For our purpose we can look at retinol-containing creams and retinoic acid-containing creams such as tretinoin, which is the active form. Retinol has a milder effect because it has to be converted to retinoic acid in the skin. Retinoids are the only topical substance that have a receptor on the nucleus of cells. So once applied onto the skin, they will actually penetrate the cells and bind to the nucleus receptors. This allows retinoids to have a direct effect on the DNA of the cells.

These substances are used to treat acne, sun damage, pigmentation, and have a very powerful anti-ageing effect. Generally speaking, they have an effect on the five major cells in the skin. They force the keratinocytes to grow faster and speed up the epidermal cycle. This initially causes dryness and peeling on the surface of the skin, which most people dislike. However, this side effect is temporary and will subside as the dead corneocytes are exfoliated. The end result is healthy youthful corneocytes at the surface.

They also reduce excess oil in the skin by having an effect on the pilosebaceous unit. This also helps to shrink the pores and of course improve acne as well. The side effect is temporary dryness, which can be alleviated by applying a light oil-free moisturizer. However, once the skin's internal hydration is restored, it will no longer feel dry as it is now healthy from the inside out. The third effect is on the fibroblasts. Fibroblasts are directly activated and prompted to create more collagen, elastin, and hyaluronic acid, which will result in thickening of the dermis and improved skin elasticity and hydration. There is also an effect on the blood vessels in the skin. There is more blood, thus more nutrients and oxygen in the skin. This can cause temporary redness and flushing in the skin, which again will subside with continuous use. Finally the fifth effect is on the melanocytes, where pigment formation is reduced and regulated.

As you can see, retinoid-containing products are very popular and very effective, both as a prep product but also as a maintenance product. Retinoids are always best used at nighttime as they are sun-sensitive, but they also sensitize the skin to UV light, so using a UV screen during the day is an absolute must when using retinoids. Retinoids can also be combined with other agents such as AHAs or hydroquinone, which we will discuss further on.

Always remember to recommend stopping use of any retinoid about five days before a peel to stop the skin being super sensitive to the peel. Also remember that if the patient's skin has been prepared with retinoids, it will absorb much more of the acid and the peel will be deeper. So be very careful with this. Please make sure that you follow the manufacturer's advice. Also it is important to stop the use of retinoids during pregnancy and breast feeding.

I always try to incorporate at least one retinoid-containing product in the patient's skincare routine as I know that this will transform their skin. And if you are selling them a retinoid, make absolutely sure you also sell them a good sunscreen at the same time.

Bakuchiol

Bakuchiol is not a very well-known ingredient; however, it has an effect similar to retinoids but is much milder, without the erythema and peeling. It can also be used both during the day and at nighttime and is safe to use during pregnancy and breast feeding. So it's an excellent alternative for those who wish to have a more gentle approach or those who for some reason are unable to use a retinoid.

Hydroquinone (10,11)

There are many ingredients with an anti-tyrosinase activity; however, hydroquinone (HQ) is the most powerful of all. HQ stops the melanocytes from producing melanin, but this process is totally reversible. A lot of medical practitioners are worried or even scared of using HQ, because they have heard it could cause cancer or cause horrible side effects. Yes, HQ is just like tretinoin – a prescription drug – and yes, it has to be used with caution, but it is very useful and can be used safely to manage pigmentation disorders. HQ is best used at 2–4%. Concentrations of higher than 4% are not recommended as they can cause side effects. Generally HQ causes erythema, dryness, peeling, and some minor irritation but that will subside and doesn't last.

HQ is often used in conjunction with a retinoid to enhance the effect of lightening and reducing skin pigmentation. Just like retinoids, HQ is not suitable during pregnancy and breast feeding, so a non-HQ anti-tyrosinase product would be preferred then. The correct dosage of HQ is twice daily to treat pigmentation, and it is best to gradually reduce the dose to once daily and then once every other day rather than stopping it abruptly. Again, use of a sunscreen is mandatory when using HQ. Excessive use of HQ and prolonged use of it at high percentage could result in dyschromias and exogenous ochronosis, which is a type of hyperpigmentation in itself and rather difficult to treat.

HQ is safe under medical supervision and at 2–4% with intervals of reduced use as per medical advice. It is very useful to treat pigmentation disorders such as melasma and excellent to use as a skin prep tool in darker skin types and also very effective at treating side effects such as PIH. Always ensure that any active ingredients such as retinoids, HQ, or strong AHAs are stopped about five days before any peel to avoid the risk of going too deep.

Cysteamine (12–17)

Cysteamine is a relatively new component that allows us to treat hyperpigmentation without using hydroquinone-based products. Some patients may prefer not to use hydroquinone or may actually be allergic to it. In this case cysteamine offers a good alternative. Cysteamine cream contains cysteamine hydrochloride, a metabolite of L-cysteine, and a natural cellular component. L-cysteamine inhibits melanin synthesis.

The cream is applied to the pigmented skin areas once daily. It is washed off after 15 minutes. To reduce irritation, it should be applied at least an hour after washing the skin. After six weeks of application, the exposure time can be increased gradually if there are no signs of skin irritation such as redness or dryness. A reduction in pigmentation can be visible after six weeks. Optimal results can be obtained after 8 to 12 weeks. To maintain its effects, cysteamine cream should be continued twice weekly indefinitely.

Figure 5.2 shows a patient who had an allergic reaction and outbreak after use of hydroquinone. Some individuals can unfortunately be allergic to this ingredient. The after picture is after two weeks of using a cysteamine-based routine.

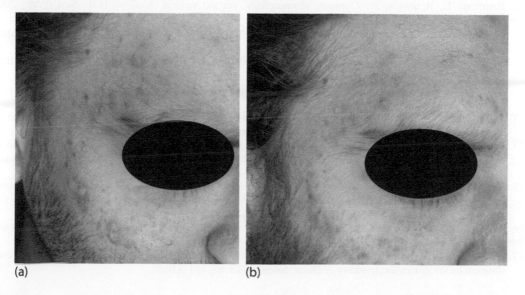

(a)   (b)

FIGURE 5.2   (a) Allergic reaction after use of hydroquinone; (b) after two weeks of cysteamine-based routine.

THE FINGERTIP UNIT

I actually dislike terms such as a pea size, half a pea size, hazelnut size, and any other vague descriptions of how much product one should use on the face.

The fingertip unit (FTU) is a much better system that allows consistent delivery of specific amounts of products onto the face. An FTU is the amount of cream that would be applied as a single continuous line of cream on the full length of the distal phalanx of a finger. This is a much better way of measuring products being applied to get a consistent result. It is especially useful for ingredients of medical grade such as tretinoin, HQ, AHA creams, etc.

REFERENCES

1. Deprez P, Pre-peel care, in: *Textbook of chemical peels*, second edition, CRC Press, Boca Raton, 2016: 7–12.
2. Obagi ZE, Skin health: The concepts, in: *Skin health restoration and rejuvenation*, Springer, New York, 2000: 27–46.
3. Baumann L, Sunscreens, in: *Cosmetic dermatology*, second edition, McGraw-Hill, New York, 2009: 245–255.
4. Baumann L, Depigmenting agents, antioxidants, in: *Cosmetic dermatology*, second edition, McGraw-Hill, New York, 2009: 284–286.
5. Baumann L, Antioxidants, in: *Cosmetic dermatology*, second edition, McGraw-Hill, New York, 2009: 292–311.
6. Obagi ZE, Alpha hydroxy acids, in: *Skin health restoration and rejuvenation*, Springer, New York, 2000: 53–56.
7. Obagi ZE, Tretinoin, in: *Skin health restoration and rejuvenation*, Springer, New York, 2000: 48–52.
8. Deprez P, Tretinoin, in: *Textbook of chemical peels*, second edition, CRC Press, Boca Raton, 2016: 8–9.
9. Baumann L, Retinoids, in: *Cosmetic dermatology*, second edition, McGraw-Hill, New York, 2009: 256–262.
10. Obagi ZE, Hydroquinone and other depigmenting agents, in: *Skin health restoration and rejuvenation*, Ringer, New York, 2000: 57–63.
11. Baumann L, Depigmenting agents, Tyrosinase inhibitors, in: *Cosmetic dermatology*, second edition, McGraw-Hill, New York, 2009: 279–282.
12. Mahrous M, Cysteamine cream, in: *Dermnet*, April 2017: https://dermnetnz.org/topics/cysteamine-cream accessed 24/1/2023.
13. Qiu L, Zhang M, Sturm RA, Gardiner B, Tonks I, Kay G, Parsons PG, Inhibition of melanin synthesis by cysteamine in human melanoma cells. *Journal of Investigative Dermatology* 2000 Jan; 114 (1): 21–7.
14. Mansouri P, Farshi S, Hashemi Z, Kasraee B, Evaluation of the efficacy of cysteamine 5% cream in the treatment of epidermal melasma: A randomized double-blind placebo-controlled trial. *British Journal of Dermatology* 2018; 173 (1): 209–217.
15. Farshi A, Mansouri P, Kasraee B, Efficacy of cysteamine cream in the treatment of epidermal melasma, evaluating by Dermacatch as a new measurement method: A randomized double blind placebo controlled study. *Journal of Dermatological Treatment* 2017; 29(2): 1–8.
16. Kasraee B, Deodorized cysteamine* as a depigmenting agent for the treatment of melasma. Pigment Cell Melanoma Research 2017; 30: e27–e137.
17. Hsu C, Mahdi HA, Pourmahdi M, Ahmadi S, Cysteamine cream as a new skin depigmenting product. *Journal of the American Academy of Dermatology* 2013; 68: 4–1 AB189.

Investigations and Peri-Operative Measures

6

Chapter 7 concerns general contra-indications for peels, which apply to all three categories of peel.

For **superficial peels** no specific investigations are required: just check the medical history (of course) and be aware of the Fitzpatrick skin type.

For **medium peels**, again specific no investigations are required. Always ask about any history of herpes simplex and cover the patient with anti-virals for five to seven days.

For a **deep peel** anti-virals are a must for two weeks. I would also recommend prophylactic antibiotic cover for a full-face deep peel (and probably also best for mosaic peels).

For a full-face deep peel I would also recommend a blood test analysis prior to the peel. I usually test for full blood count (FBC), kidney and liver function (U&Es and LFTs) and if any doubt also fasting glucose and hepatitis C serology.

A full-face Botulinum Toxin treatment should be carried out one to two weeks before a deep peel. It should treat the full upper face (glabella, frontalis, and peri-orbital) and sometimes even hypermobile areas of the lower face (DAOs and orbicularis oris). This is to ensure that the expressive muscles of the face are as calm as possible during the first few months following the peel so that as many wrinkles as possible can be reduced.

I do not perform full-face deep peels on anyone who has cardiac, renal, or hepatic illness history; also, a previous history of diabetes or hepatitis C is not acceptable. An ECG is only really required if there is any doubt about cardiac health, which the patient should already have disclosed at the consultation.

The question is, is cardiac monitoring necessary during a deep peel? We know from years of experience by various authors that cardiac arrhythmia is very rare even with full-face deep peels when general anaesthesia is not used. Indeed, with our modern formulations and protocols that combine good analgesia with localized anaesthesia, arrhythmia is rarely seen.

For localized deep peels in mosaic peels I do not worry about cardiac monitoring.

For full-face deep phenol peels I do monitor the blood oxygen saturation and pulse with a fingertip oxygen saturation meter device and I also monitor the blood pressure before and during the peel. I monitor the heart rhythm with a small cardiac monitor that can look at the rhythm at any time required. I also make sure I have IV access and I provide intravenous fluids during the peel (usually 500 ml to 1 L of normal saline, very slowly during the procedure), in which further analgesia can be mixed (1).

A typical list of medication needed for a phenol peel before, during, and after the peel would consist of:

Antivirals: aciclovir

To be taken two days before and up to 12 days after the peel (**one** tablet, **five times** every day)

DOI: 10.1201/9781003244134-6

TABLE 6.1 Roster of list of medication taken day by day from day -2 to day 12 for a phenol peel. PRN: take these drugs only if needed.

	DAY -2	DAY -1	DAY 0 PEEL	DAY 1	DAY 2	DAY 3	DAY 4	DAY 5	DAY 6	DAY 7	DAY 8	DAY 9	DAY 10	DAY 11	DAY 12
Aciclovir (antiviral) 5x daily															
Alprazolam (calming) 1x night		PRN													
Co-codamol (painkillers) 2x4 daily				PRN	PRN	PRN									
Antibiotics 1x4 daily															
Hydroxyzine (antihistamines) 2x daily															

Anxiolytics: alprazolam
One tablet the night before the peel and up to three days after the peel

Antihistamine: hydroxyzine hydrochloride
For four days starting after the treatment

Analgesics: co-codamol
For four days starting the following day after the peel

Antibiotics: flucloxacillin
For seven days, starting on the second day following the peel

Artificial tear drops
As needed

Bepanthene ointment
One tube and Vaseline ointment one tube

Fucidine ointment
One tube (topical antibiotic)

Table 6.1 sets out the information I give to the patients to make it even easier for them.

REFERENCE

1. Deprez P, Phenol: Toxicity, causes, prevention and treatment, in: *Textbook of chemical peels*, second edition, CRC Press, Boca Raton, 2017: 230–238.

Peeling Procedures

7

The ideal patients are healthy individuals.

The general list of contra-indications for any peel is:

- Patients who are pregnant or breast-feeding
- A history of keloid or hypertrophic scarring
- Severe auto-immune illnesses
- Skin collagen diseases (for example, Ehlers Danlos syndrome)
- Skin infections
- Active cold sores
- Dark skin types, unless appropriate peel is chosen and anti-tyrosinase products are used
- Cancers under treatment including radiotherapy
- Recent surgery such as face-lifts in the last six months
- Oral Isotretinoin (Roaccutane) in the last 6–12 months

For a phenol peel there are the following additional contra-indications:

- Patients who use IMAO antidepressants
- Insulin dependent diabetes
- Disease and arrhythmia
- Kidney disease
- Liver disease
- Severe respiratory illnesses
- Severe anxiety and or claustrophobia
- A low pain threshold
- Use of a lot of analgesia of any kind

There are many different peeling brands available on the market. I have personally worked with several of them. The products mentioned in this book are those I use myself in my practice. This does not mean that other brands are in any way inferior; these are just what I have used for a long time and find work for me.

> The products mentioned in this text are:
>
> **Neostrata glycolic peels for AHA**
> **Obagi Blue peel radiance for BHA**
> **SkinTech Easy TCA and Easy TCA Pain Control for 15% TCA**
> **SkinTech Unideep for 25% TCA**
> **SkinTech Easy Phen Light for 30% phenol**
> **SkinTech Lip & Eyelid Formula for 60% phenol**

DOI: 10.1201/9781003244134-7

AHA AND BHA PEELS

There are quite a few different AHAs that are used in skincare ingredients and also as peeling substances. AHAs are hydrophilic, whereas BHA is lipophilic. AHAs penetrate through the epidermis by reducing the corneocyte adhesion. Their molecules are small enough to get through the very small intercellular gaps in the epidermis. Glycolic acid has the smallest molecule size and can therefore penetrate faster and deeper compared to other AHAs. Various AHAs have slightly different effects on the skin and therefore very often they can be combined with each other (1).

Commonly Used AHAs

The most commonly used AHAs are as follows:

Glycolic acid

Glycolic acid is the smallest AHA molecule; therefore it penetrates faster through the gaps between the corneocytes and keratinocytes. It is widely used in many skincare formulations and also in various chemical peels. It exfoliates the skin, helps to improve sun damage, enhances hyaluronic acid and collagen levels in the skin, and improves skin pigmentation. Like all AHAs, two factors determine the strength of this peeling agent. One is the percentage and the other is the PH of the formula.

Lactic acid

Lactic acid has a slightly larger molecule so penetrates a bit more slowly. It is the next shortest AHA molecule after glycolic acid, so at the same percentages it destroys the epidermis more slowly. It also has an anti-tyrosinase activity so is great to use in formulations for pigmentation.

Other AHAs

Many other AHA combinations are used as they each have a slightly different activity.

Ascorbic acid or Vitamin C is an AHA derivative which has been shown to stimulate collagen production and reduce melanin production. It acts as a free radical scavenger and is classified as an antioxidant.

Citric acid has a larger molecule size than glycolic acid. It has a similar action but penetrates more slowly and it is meant to even out the skin colour and pigmentation.

Mandelic acid again has a large molecule size. It has a specific activity on oily skin and acne-prone skin.

Azelaic acid has an anti-pigmentation effect and also works well in acne.

Phytic acid also has an anti-tyrosinase activity.

Kojic acid also has a strong anti-tyrosinase activity so is often used in formulations for pigmentation.

Peeling Procedure with AHAs

Always follow the protocols and instructions of the specific peel you are using according to the manufacturer's advice and your training.

1) Remove all makeup and cleanse the skin.
2) Cleanse the skin again with your specific pre-peel cleanser.
3) Dry the skin off.
4) Protect sensitive areas of the face such as the peri-orbital area, nasal creases, corners of the mouth, etc. with some Vaseline and possibly also cover the eyes with cotton pads.
5) Take out the required amount of your AHA peel into a small dish or bowl.
6) Use a fan brush for the peel. Wet the brush thoroughly and make sure you take off any excess. You do not want the peel to drip off the face or go into the hairline. Some gel-based formulations are more practical than fully liquid formulations.
7) Apply the peel in an even layer onto the forehead, nose, chin, top lip, and finally cheek areas. Stay well away from the peri-orbital area.
8) Once the full face has been covered, start a timer. The peel can stay on the skin for the maximum length of time determined by the specific manufacturer. Do not exceed this time to keep the peel safe. Remember AHAs are designed to be superficial, and if they penetrate too deeply, they can cause complications.
9) The expected reaction on the face is erythema and nothing further.
10) Once the time is up, start neutralizing the peel with your neutralizer (if that is recommended; some AHA peels do not require neutralization, but generally most do). Either rub or brush or spray on the neutralizer until all the acid has been neutralized. Some neutralizers cause foaming when mixed with acid, so once no further foam is noticed the process has been successful. Other neutralizers change colour as they neutralize the acid, so please refer to the individual peel protocols you are using.
11) Remove all residue off the face with wet cotton pads or gauze swabs. Make sure the face is thoroughly cleansed with water.
12) Apply the recommended post-peel recovery cream and sunblock if required.
13) Give aftercare instructions to the patient.

Figure 7.1 shows the typical required equipment for an AHA peel (in this case, a 70% Neostrata glycolic acid peel). We have the pre-peel cleanser, some gauze swabs, the acid itself dispensed in a small container, gloves, a fan brush, and the neutralizer.

Figure 7.2 shows the process of simply cleansing the skin with a cleanser and water.

Figure 7.3 shows the next step which is preparing the skin with a pre-peel cleanser.

Figure 7.4 shows the eyes being protected with some cotton pads. Any delicate areas may now be covered in a little bit of Vaseline.

Figure 7.5 shows selection of the peel (50% glycolic acid) to apply.

Figure 7.6 shows application of the peel with a fan brush.

Figure 7.7 shows timing of the peel. Remember that AHA peels are time-dependent, so you will need to time the duration of action (in this case, three minutes).

Figure 7.8 shows starting the neutralization process which has to be done to remove the active acid from the face.

Figure 7.9 shows the foaming reaction of the neutralizer mixing with the acid. We keep neutralizing until there is no further white foam. Please remember this is specific to Neostrata; in other systems this reaction may not happen or they might change colour as the acid is neutralized.

Figure 7.10 shows washing off the neutralizer.

Figure 7.11 shows the final step – application of some SPF.

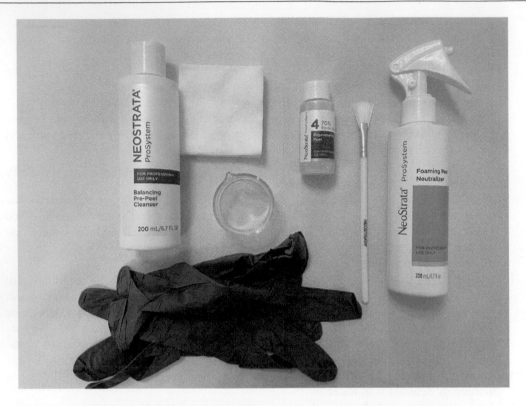

FIGURE 7.1   Equipment needed for an AHA peel.

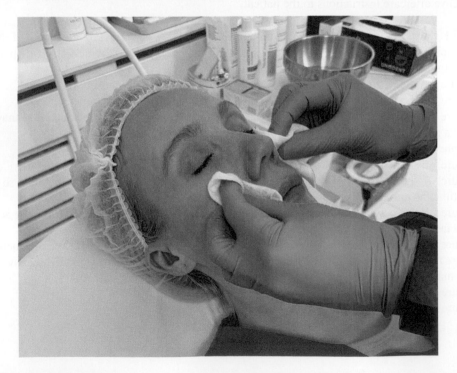

FIGURE 7.2   Cleansing the skin.

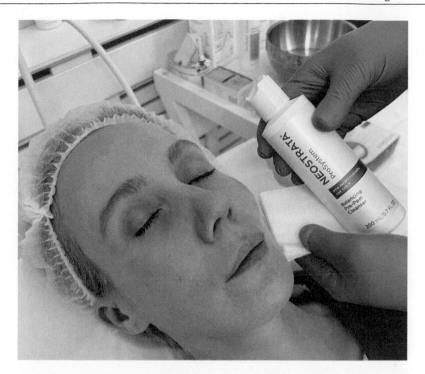

FIGURE 7.3 Preparing the skin with pre-peel cleanser.

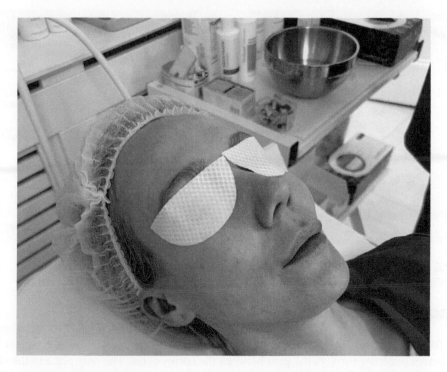

FIGURE 7.4 Protection for the eyes.

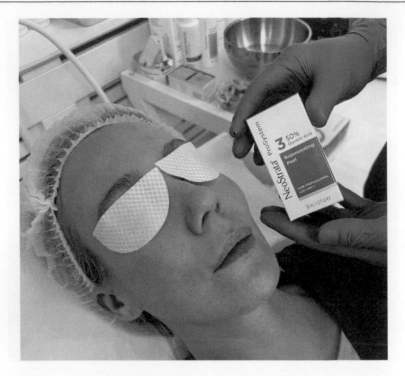

FIGURE 7.5 Selecting the peel to apply.

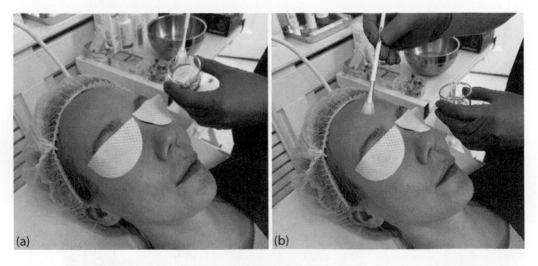

(a)   (b)

FIGURE 7.6 (a, b) Applying the peel with a fan brush.

Commonly Used BHAs

The only BHA used in peelings is salicylic acid. It has a much larger molecule, and as it is also lipophilic, it cannot penetrate through the gaps between the corneocytes. The only place in the skin where it can penetrate is the pilosebaceous unit. Salicylic acid is a natural anti-inflammatory, so this makes

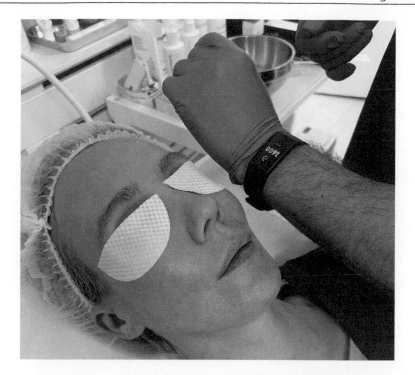

FIGURE 7.7   Timing the peel.

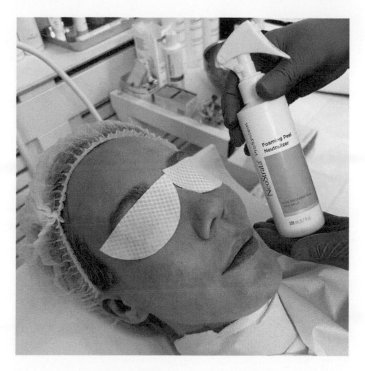

FIGURE 7.8   Starting the neutralization process.

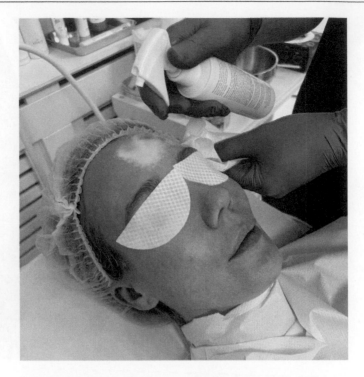

FIGURE 7.9 Foaming reaction as neutralizer mixes with the acid.

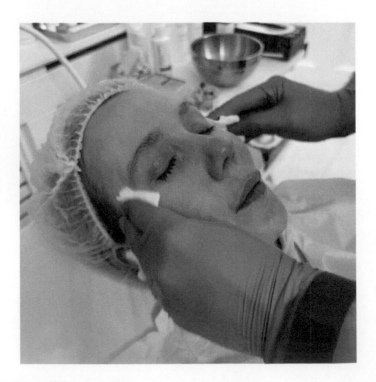

FIGURE 7.10 Washing off the neutralizer.

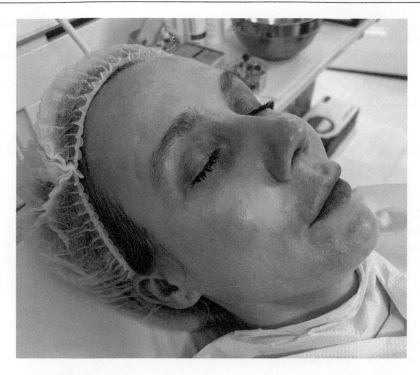

FIGURE 7.11   Application of SPF.

this agent perfect to use for oily skin types and acne-prone skin. Sometimes AHAs and BHA are combined in peels to get the benefit of both types of acids.

Peeling Procedure with BHA

Always follow the protocols and instructions of the specific peel you are using according to the manufacturer's advice and your training.

1) Remove all makeup and cleanse the skin.
2) Cleanse the skin again with your specific pre-peel cleanser.
3) Dry the skin off.
4) Some peels require a pre-peel toner. Refer to the specific peel protocols.
5) Take out the required amount of your BHA peel into a small dish or bowl.
6) Use a fan brush or a gauze swab for the peel according to the protocol. Wet the brush or swab thoroughly and make sure you take off any excess. You do not want the peel to drip off the face or go into the hairline.
7) Apply the peel in an even layer onto the forehead, nose, chin, top lip, and finally cheek areas. Stay well away from the peri-orbital area.
8) Once the full face has been covered, start a timer if this is required according to protocol. The peel can stay on the skin for the maximum length of time determined by the specific manufacturer. Do not exceed this time to keep the peel safe. Remember that BHAs are designed to be superficial, and if they penetrate too deeply, they can cause complications.
9) Salicylic acid generally causes a pseudo-frost on the face. This is just crystallization of the acid on the skin as it dries.

10) Once the time is up or the pseudo-frost has appeared, start removing the acid with water-soaked gauze swabs or cotton pads according to your protocol.
11) Remove all further residue off the face with wet cotton pads or gauze swabs. Make sure the face is thoroughly cleansed with water.
12) Apply the recommended post-peel recovery cream and sunblock if required.
13) Give aftercare instructions to the patient.

Figure 7.12 shows the required equipment for – in this instance – an Obagi Blue peel Radiance, which is based on salicylic acid. We need the pre-peel solution, the acid itself, some gauze swabs, and some gloves.

Figure 7.13 shows cleansing the skin with a cleanser and water.

Figure 7.14 shows the next step of applying the prep solution with some gauze swabs.

Figure 7.15 shows preparing the acid to be applied.

Figure 7.16 shows the gauze swab soaked in the acid being rubbed on the face to apply the peeling solution all over, except the eyelids and the area too close to the mouth.

Figure 7.17 shows the pseudo-frosting of BHA forming on the skin; remember this is not a true frost, but just the salicylic acid crystals on the skin.

Figure 7.18 shows the cleansing of the leftovers of the product with just simple water.

Figure 7.19 shows the endpoint, which is application of an SPF to finish the peel.

Figure 7.20 shows the desquamation after a few days with an AHA-BHA combination peel. Downtime is only a couple of days of dry flaky skin. The peri-oral area is usually the first area to peel off with any peels due to the natural movement of the mouth.

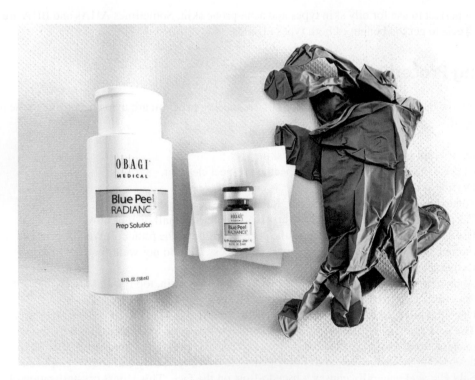

FIGURE 7.12   Equipment needed for a BHA peel.

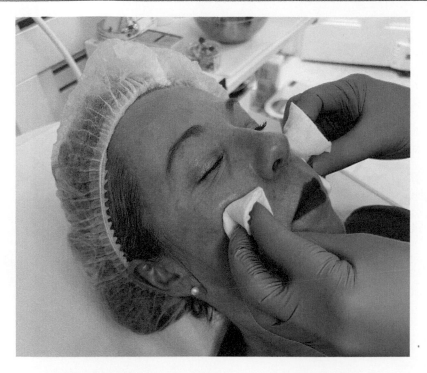

FIGURE 7.13   Cleansing the skin with cleanser and water.

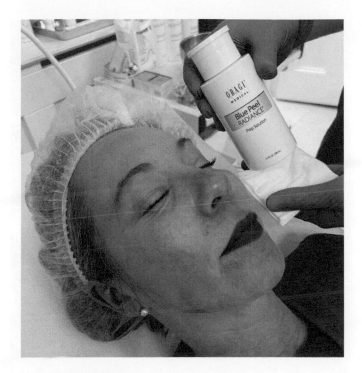

FIGURE 7.14   Applying the prep solution.

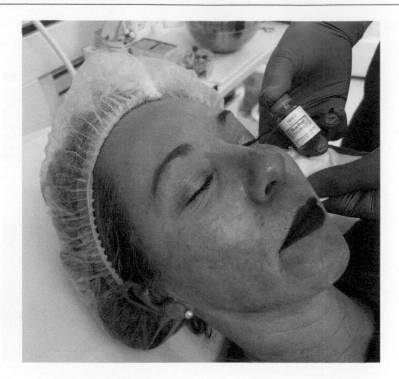

FIGURE 7.15 Preparing the acid.

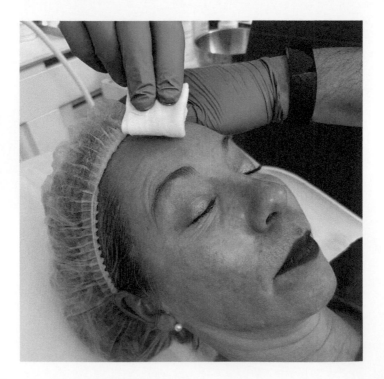

FIGURE 7.16 Gauze swab being applied to the face.

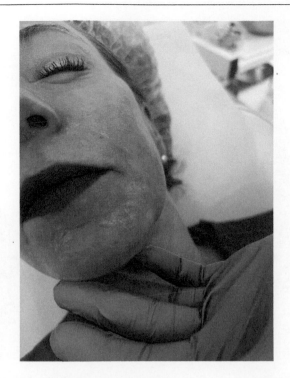

FIGURE 7.17   Pseudo-frosting of BHA forming on the skin.

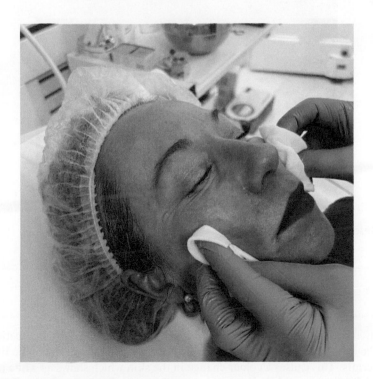

FIGURE 7.18   Cleansing leftover product with water.

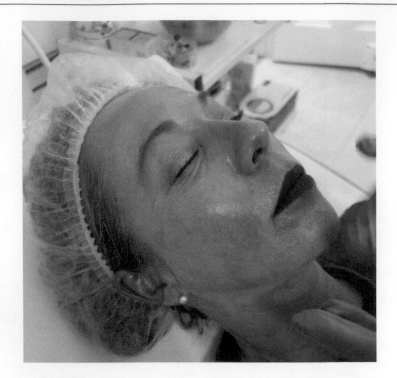

FIGURE 7.19   Applying an SPF.

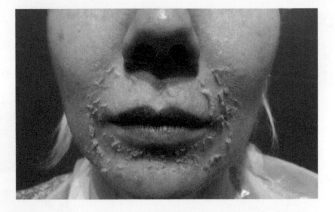

FIGURE 7.20   Desquamation a few days after an AHA-BHA combination peel.

TCA

The mode of action of TCA is completely different to AHAs and BHA. Trichloracetic acid denatures the proteins in the cells as it comes in contact with them. It essentially destroys the living cells of the epidermis and dermis. This causes a colour change in the skin which shows as white areas on the skin called frosting (2,3). Skin re-epithelializes with a week and replaces damaged cells by healthy cells, and this process also causes a lot of new collagen growth in the dermis.

It is worth mentioning that the percentage of TCA only really refers to the speed of acid penetration into the skin. So, for example, a 10% TCA gives a superficial peel; however, multiple coats of application of the same acid can produce a medium or even a deep peel. A 35% TCA would penetrate faster, so one or two coats will give a medium-depth peel.

I personally prefer the multi-layer approach – for example, with a 15 or 20% TCA solution. This can also give perfect medium peels but allows the practitioner more control as with each layer the acid penetrates deeper and it allows the practitioner to assess the depth of the peel. This of course will increase the safety of the procedure. (I will explain further below how to assess the peel depth while performing it.) (4,5,6)

For TCA to be applied evenly to the entire face, the face has to be divided into cosmetic subunits. Figure 7.21 shows how to do that.

Peeling Procedure for Superficial TCA Peels

1) Remove all makeup and cleanse the skin.
2) Cleanse the skin again with your specific pre-peel cleanser.
3) Dry the skin off.
4) Take out the required amount of your TCA peel into a small dish or bowl. Some formulations require mixing, while others don't. If mixing TCA with a base solution is required, make absolutely sure that you follow the exact instructions of the brand you use to get the correct percentage of the TCA after mixing. Three good examples of TCA peels that need mixing with a base solution are SkinTech Easy TCA and Easy TCA Pain Control and also the Obagi Blue peel.

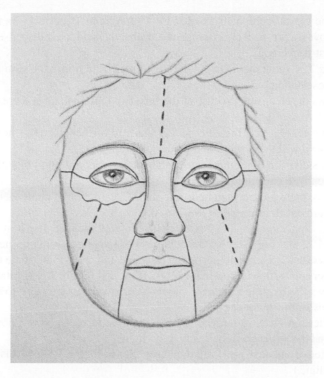

FIGURE 7.21 Division of the face in cosmetic subunits. The forehead and temple area is divided into two sections. The cheeks are divided into a lateral and medial section. The nose is a separate area. The top lip and lower lip/chin area form the peri-oral area. The upper and lower eyelids form the peri-orbital area.

5) Use one or two cotton buds to apply the TCA solution to the face. Make absolutely sure that the cotton buds are not too wet so that the TCA does not drip and run down the face or, even worse, into the eyes – *this would be extremely dangerous.*

The face is usually divided into multiple cosmetic subunits, and the TCA is meticulously applied to the skin in an even layer. Once one area is fully covered, then move on to the next area and move around the face to complete the application in all areas.

6) Use a fan to dry the TCA on the skin and cool the face off. TCA application causes stinging and heat and can be quite uncomfortable even at low percentages.

7) There is no need to use a timer as most TCA peels are self-neutralizing, and there is no need to remove them. There are, however, exceptions to this rule, so please make sure you follow the instructions according to your specific peel.

8) The expected reaction on the face is first erythema and then frosting. For a superficial TCA peel we expect to see frosting points, which are very small white dots on the skin sometimes only as big as the tip of a needle. The appearance of frosting points indicates that the acid has penetrated the basal layer of the epidermis.

9) If frosting does not appear or a deeper frosting is desired, then apply a second coat to all the areas of the face as before and dry and cool off the face with a fan.

10) The next level of frosting is when the points start merging and start covering larger areas of the face. This level of frosting is called frosting clouds. This indicates that the TCA has now penetrated the Grenz zone just below the basal layer. This is the deepest level for a superficial TCA peel.

11) Apply the recommended post-peel recovery cream and sunblock if required.

12) Give aftercare instructions to the patient.

Figure 7.22 shows the typical equipment needed for a superficial TCA peel – in this case, a SkinTech TCA peel – some gloves, a pre-peel cleanser, gauze swabs, the acid itself dispensed in a container, cotton buds, and the post-peel cream.

Figures 7.23 and 7.24 show the different depths of penetration into the skin in the schematic diagram and clinical presentation.

Figure 7.25 shows the cleansing process of the face from all makeup and creams to get the patient ready for the peel.

Figure 7.26 shows use of a SkinTech pre-peel cleanser to further clean the face again. The more we clean, the better the acid will do its work and penetrate evenly.

Figure 7.27 shows division of the face into small sections according to Fig. 21 so that the peel can be applied systematically to each area.

Figure 7.28 shows dipping the cotton buds into the TCA solution to make them wet. It is important that the cotton buds are **not dripping and not too wet**.

Figure 7.29 shows application of TCA to the first section of the face. It is best to use circular movements to apply the TCA, making sure that the acid has been applied evenly to the entire area.

Figure 7.30 shows some frosting points on the forehead and cheeks and some frosting clouds on the nose and glabella after application of one coat of 15% TCA, and Figure 7.31 similarly shows the cheeks.

Figure 7.32 shows the frosting confluent clouds after two coats of TCA 15% on the cheeks, and Figure 7.33 shows this similarly for the full face.

During the application phase, a fan was used to cool the face off. Now a post-peel cream will be applied to the face and the patient will be ready to go home.

(For an illustration of the post-peel cream, please refer to Figure 7.52, as this patient had a further coat of TCA in the clinic.)

The peel is now completed and the patient is ready to go home.

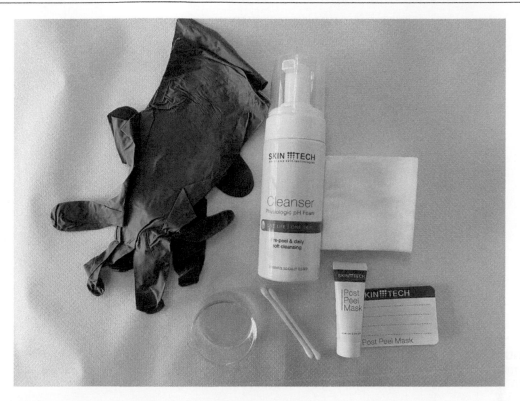

FIGURE 7.22 Equipment needed for a superficial TCA peel.

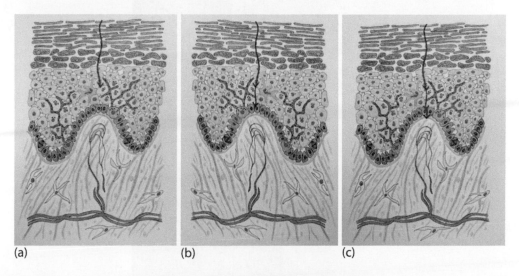

(a)   (b)   (c)

FIGURE 7.23 TCA penetration into the different depths of the skin: (a) Intra-epidermal TCA would most likely just cause some erythema. (b) Once TCA reaches the basal layer, frosting points will appear on the skin. (c) The final stage of a superficial TCA peel is penetration into the Grenz zone, which would show itself as frosting clouds.

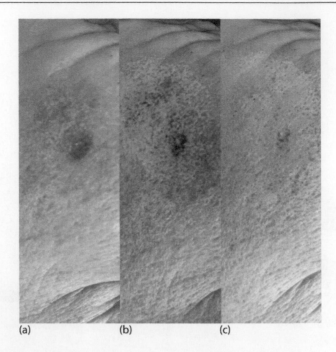

(a)   (b)   (c)

FIGURE 7.24   The three stages of frosting on the same area of skin: (a) frosting points; (b) frosting clouds; (c) fuller white frost with a pink background ('pink frost'). In this patient with oily skin one more coat of 15% TCA would be required to get a proper medium-depth frost.

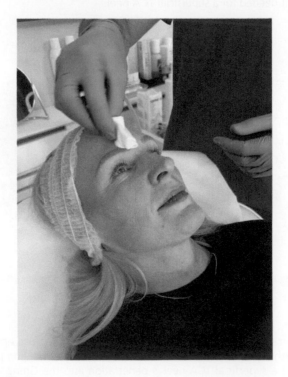

FIGURE 7.25   Cleansing the face.

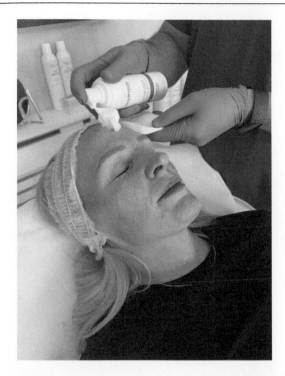

FIGURE 7.26 Using a SkinTech pre-peel cleanser.

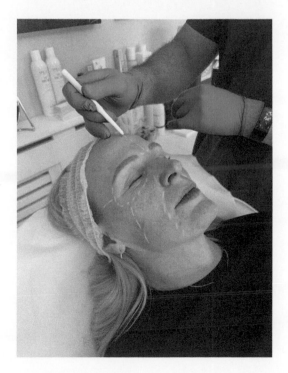

FIGURE 7.27 Dividing the face into small sections.

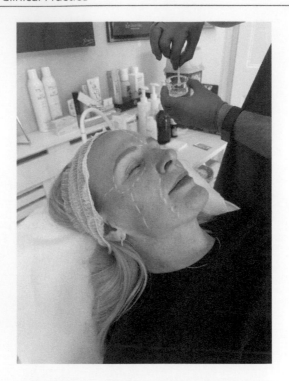

FIGURE 7.28   Wetting the cotton buds.

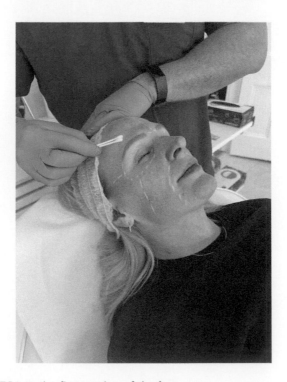

FIGURE 7.29   Applying TCA to the first section of the face.

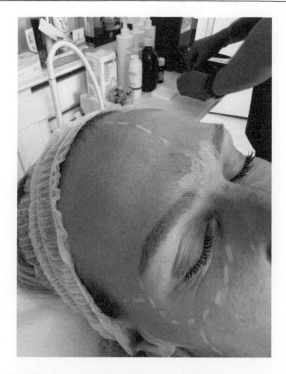

FIGURE 7.30 Frosting points after application of one coat of TCA.

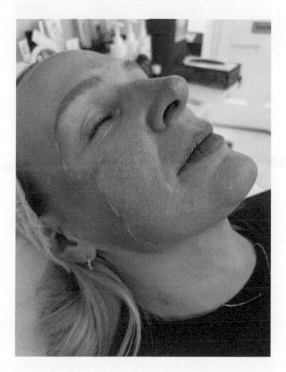

FIGURE 7.31 Frosting points on the cheeks after one coat of 15% TCA.

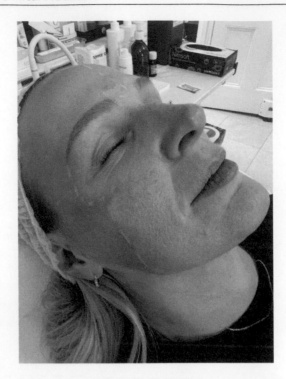

FIGURE 7.32   Frosting confluent clouds on the cheeks after two coats of TCA.

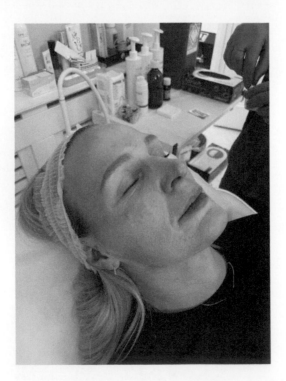

FIGURE 7.33   Confluent frosting clouds on the entire face after two coats of TCA 15% on the full face. One or two coats (depending on skin type and skin prep) are enough to give a nice superficial TCA peel to the Grenz Zone.

Figure 7.34 shows a typical example of the application of TCA using two cotton buds. Having two cotton buds gives more strength to the applicator compared to one cotton bud.

Figures 7.35 and 7.36 show how frosting clouds may appear on a patient with a higher skin type rating.

Peeling Procedure for Medium TCA Peels

1) Give your patient some oral analgesia 30–45 mins before the peel (for example, an NSAID and/or codeine phosphate).
2) Remove all makeup and cleanse the skin.
3) Cleanse the skin again with your specific pre-peel cleanser.

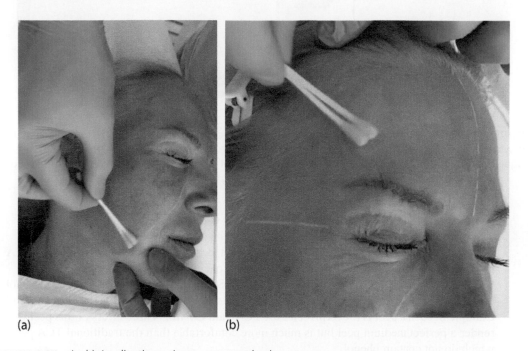

(a)   (b)

FIGURE 7.34   (a, b) Application using two cotton buds.

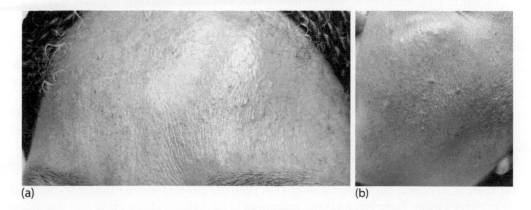

(a)   (b)

FIGURE 7.35   (a, b) Frosting clouds on the forehead and on the cheek of a patient with skin type VI.

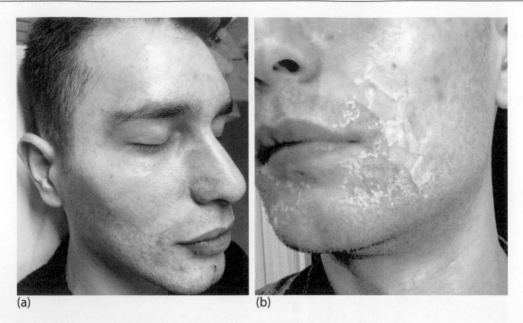

(a)   (b)

FIGURE 7.36   (a) Confluent frosting clouds after two coats of 15% TCA on the face. One more coat and this would potentially become a medium-depth TCA. (b) The same patient during the healing phase. The desquamation is much more pronounced compared to a light peel. Downtime is roughly around five days.

4) Dry the skin off.
5) Use pure alcohol to fully disinfect the skin all over with a gauze swab.
6) Then use pure acetone to fully degrease the face with a gauze swab.
7) Some practitioners prefer to do regional blocks with local anaesthesia before a medium TCA peel. This is explained further in the section about phenol peels.
   Medium TCA peels are typically quite painful. Sometimes mixtures of TCA and phenol are used to improve this discomfort, as phenol acts as an anaesthetic for the skin. A good example of such a peel is the SkinTech East TCA Pain Control. Three layers of this peel will render a perfect medium peel but is much more comfortable than the traditional TCA peels which do not contain phenol.
8) Take out the required amount of your TCA peel into a small dish or bowl. Some formulations require mixing, while others don't. If mixing TCA with a base solution is required, make absolutely sure that you follow the exact instructions of the brand you use to get the correct percentage of the TCA after mixing. Three good examples of TCA peels that need mixing with a base solution are SkinTech Easy TCA and Easy TCA Pain Control and also the Obagi Blue peel.
9) Use one or two cotton buds to apply the TCA solution to the face. Make absolutely sure that the cotton buds are not too wet so that the TCA does not drip and run down the face or even worse in the eyes – *this is extremely dangerous.*
   The face is usually divided into multiple cosmetic subunits, and the TCA is meticulously applied to the skin in an even layer. Once one area is fully covered, then move on to the next area and move around the face to complete the application in all areas.
10) Use a fan to dry the TCA on the skin and cool the face off. TCA application causes stinging and heat and can be quite uncomfortable even at low percentages.
11) There is no need to use a timer as most TCA peels are self-neutralizing and there is no need to remove them. There are, however, exceptions to this rule, so please make sure you follow the instructions according to your specific peel.

12) The expected reaction on the face is first erythema and then frosting. For a medium TCA peel we expect to see full white frosting with a pink background all over the face.

13) If frosting does not appear or a deeper frosting is desired, then apply a second coat to all the areas of the face as before and dry and cool off the face with a fan.

14) A full white frost with a pink background indicates that the TCA has penetrated the papillary dermis. The pink background indicates that the dermal blood vessels have not yet been denatured by TCA. At this stage we also notice a papery plastic-like appearance to the skin, which is called epidermal sliding. This is due to the separation of the dermo-epidermal junction. Once TCA penetrates deeper, the pink colour and the epidermal sliding will both disappear. The frost becomes pure white as the dermal blood vessels are denatured by TCA and the oedema in the dermis pretty much removes the epidermal sliding appearance.

15) Apply the recommended post-peel recovery cream and sunblock if required.

16) Give aftercare instructions to the patient.

Figure 7.37 shows what is typically needed for a medium TCA peel – in this case, a Skintech peel: some gloves, a pre-peel cleanser, gauze swabs, the acid in a small container, cotton buds, alcohol, acetone, and post-peel cream.

Figure 7.38 shows the level of TCA penetration into the papillary dermis. This will cause a white frost with a pink background (sometimes called a pink frost) with epidermal sliding.

Figure 7.39 shows the cleansing process of the face from all makeup and creams to get the patient ready for the peel.

Figure 7.40 shows use of a SkinTech pre-peel cleanser to further clean the face again. The more we clean, the better the acid will do its work and penetrate evenly.

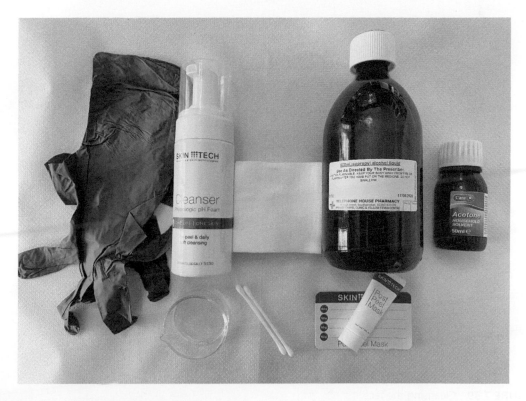

FIGURE 7.37 Equipment for a medium TCA peel.

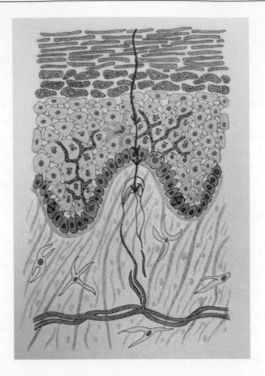

FIGURE 7.38   Level of TCA penetration into papillary dermis.

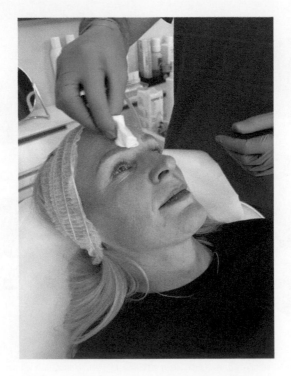

FIGURE 7.39   Cleansing the face.

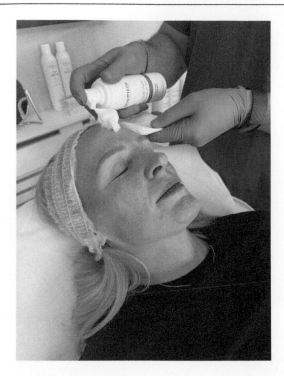

FIGURE 7.40   Using a SkinTech pre-peel cleanser.

Figure 7.41 shows use of alcohol to disinfect and totally cleanse the skin ready for a medium TCA peel.

Figure 7.42 shows the use of acetone to remove all oil from the skin and totally degrease the skin so that the TCA can penetrate even deeper into the skin.

Figure 7.43 shows division of the face into small sections according to Fig. 7.21 so that the peel can be applied systematically to each area.

Figure 7.44 shows dipping the cotton buds into the TCA solution to make them wet. **It is extremely important to make sure that the cotton buds are not dripping and not too wet**.

Figure 7.45 shows application of the TCA to the first section of the face. It is best to use circular movements to apply the TCA, making sure that the acid has been applied evenly to the entire area.

Figure 7.46 shows some frosting points on the forehead and cheeks and some frosting clouds on the nose and glabella after application of one coat of 15% TCA.

Figure 7.47 shows the frosting clouds on the cheeks after one coat of 15% TCA.

Figure 7.48 shows the frosting confluent clouds after two coats of TCA 15% on the cheeks.

Figure 7.49 shows confluent frosting clouds on the entire face after two coats of TCA 15% on the full face. One or two coats (depending on skin type and skin prep) are enough to give a nice superficial TCA peel to the Grenz Zone.

Figure 7.50 shows the face after application of three coats of TCA 15%; the eyelids have now been treated as well. The result is a uniform white frost with a pink background ('pink frost'). This is a medium-depth TCA peel and no further acid application is needed in this patient.

Using a fan during the application phase will make the patient more comfortable.

Figure 7.51 shows checking for epidermal sliding to confirm a medium TCA peel.

The peel concludes with applying post-peel cream (Figure 7.52). The patient is now ready to go home (Figure 7.53).

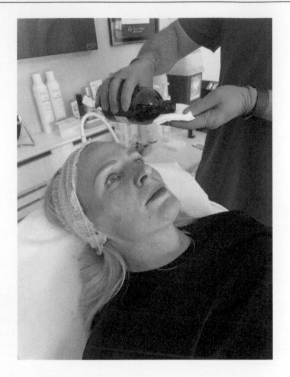

FIGURE 7.41   Using alcohol to disinfect and cleanse the skin.

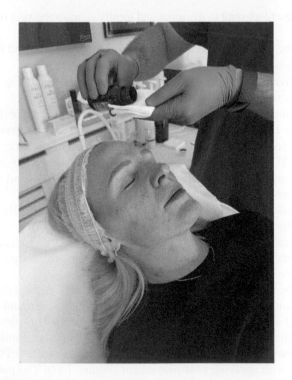

FIGURE 7.42   Using acetone to remove all oil from the skin.

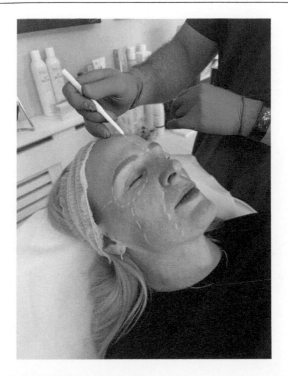

FIGURE 7.43   Division of the face into small sections.

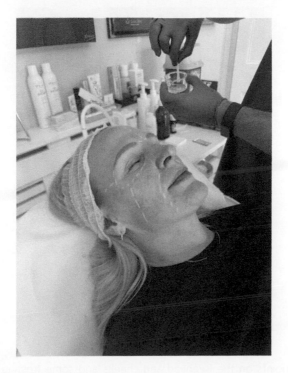

FIGURE 7.44   Dipping cotton buds into TCA.

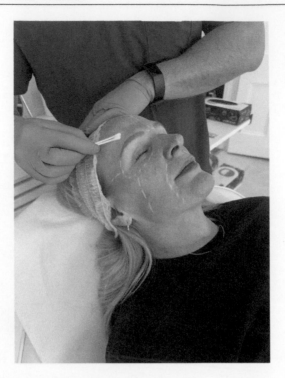

FIGURE 7.45 Applying TCA to the first section of face.

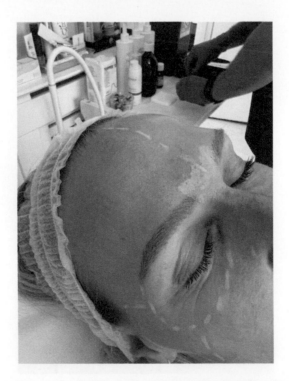

FIGURE 7.46 Frosting points on the forehead and cheeks and some frosting clouds on the nose and glabella.

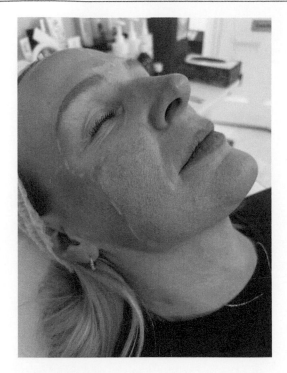

FIGURE 7.47 Frosting clouds on the cheeks.

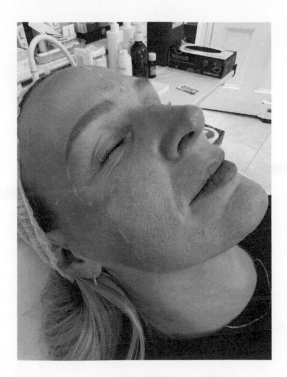

FIGURE 7.48 Frosting confluent clouds after two coats on the cheeks.

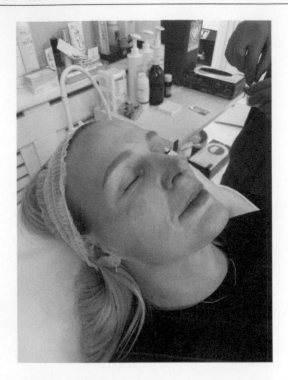

FIGURE 7.49   Confluent frosting clouds after two coats on the entire face.

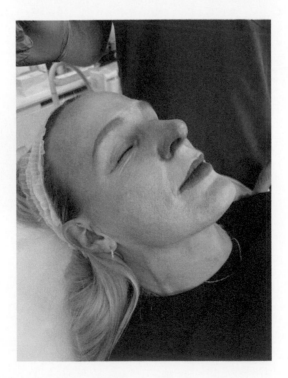

FIGURE 7.50   Pink frost after three coats of TCA.

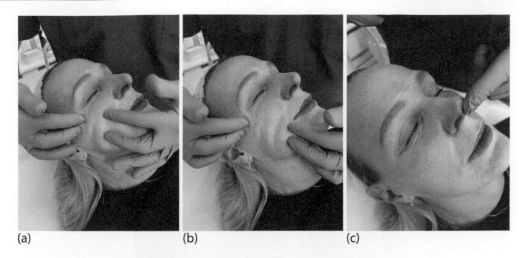

(a)   (b)   (c)

FIGURE 7.51   (a,b,c) Checking for epidermal sliding.

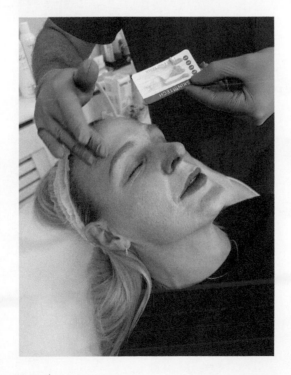

FIGURE 7.52   Applying post-peel cream.

Figure 7.54 shows the result immediately after a medium TCA with a pinkish-white frost and epidermal sliding.

Figure 7.55 shows the end point of a medium TCA peel with a pink frost and epidermal sliding, which is most visible on the lower eyelids.

Figure 7.56 shows the temporary darkening of the skin after a medium TCA peel from the day after the peel onwards in a skin type IV. This temporary darkening is normal and is not to be confused

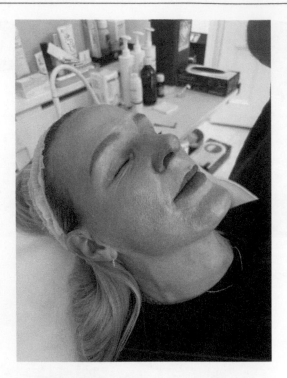

FIGURE 7.53   End of the peel after application of the post-peel cream.

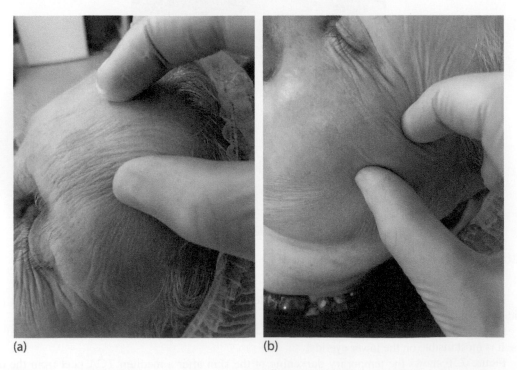

(a)   (b)

FIGURE 7.54   (a) Medium TCA peel with a pinkish white frost; (b) epidermal sliding.

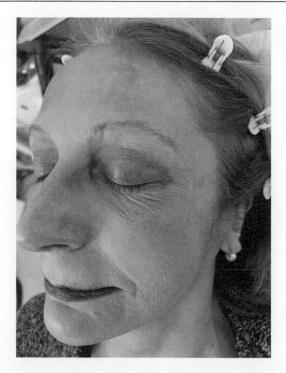

FIGURE 7.55   Medium TCA peel with a pink frost and epidermal sliding.

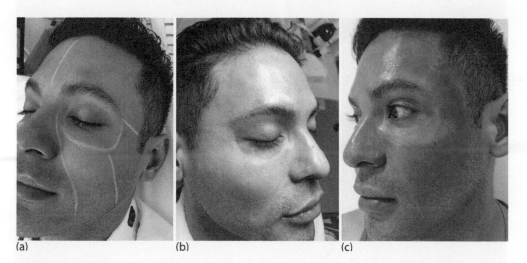

(a)   (b)   (c)

FIGURE 7.56   (a) Patient in a skin type IV marked up for medium TCA peel; (b) immediately after his medium TCA peel. The frost is not as pink as the patient naturally has more dark pigment in the skin. (c) Temporary darkening of the skin from the day after the peel onwards.

with PIH. Having said that, continued use of tyrosinase inhibitors and sun protection before and after the peel will ensure that the result remains PIH-free.

Figure 7.57 shows a typical type of desquamation on around day four to six after a medium TCA peel.

Figure 7.58 shows a patient with deep melasma on the forehead which she has had for many years. On the right side of her forehead she has even had an experimental area of deep dermabrasion many years ago that has left an odd depigmented mark in the middle of the melasma. The melasma is still

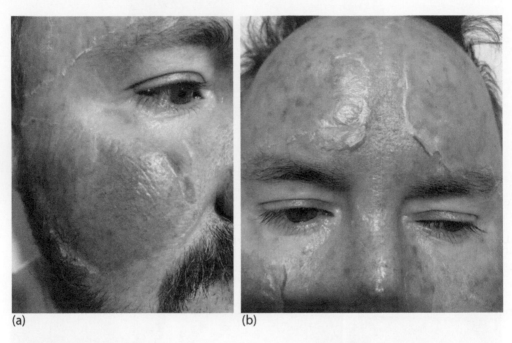

(a)   (b)

FIGURE 7.57   Typical desquamation around day four to six after a medium TCA peel.

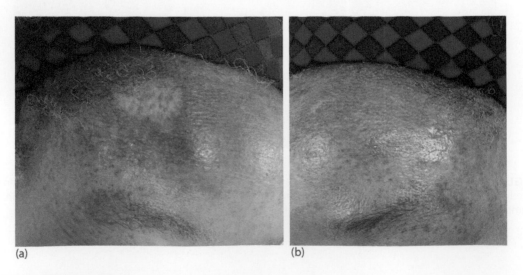

(a)   (b)

FIGURE 7.58   (a,b) Patient with deep melasma.

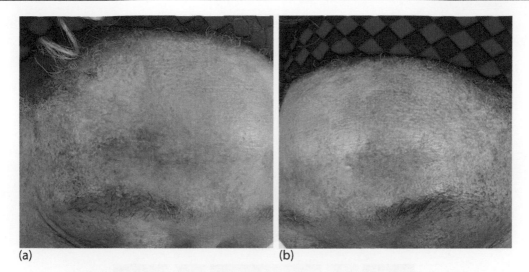

(a)   (b)

FIGURE 7.59   (a,b) Patient after a medium TCA peel.

quite noticeable despite the fact that she has been using anti-tyrosinase products for at least eight weeks. After a medium TCA peel on the forehead (Figure 7.59), the frosting is pretty uniform, but probably one more coat of 15% TCA is needed to go fully medium-depth.

Figure 7.60 shows a single medium-depth TCA treatment with three coats of 15% TCA. The patient has had a good level of improvement in her lentigines, general sun damage, and some of the fine lines; deep lines will not disappear after a medium TCA peel.

Deep TCA Peels

TCA is not indicated for the full face and can be very dangerous as it can cause extensive scarring and hypopigmentation. Deep TCA peels can be used focally to remove small lentigines or target small areas, but never the full face. A good example of a deep focal TCA peel is the SkinTech Only Touch peel. This peel penetrates deeper than the papillary dermis and a pure white frost with no pink background is expected. Immediately below the papillary dermis lies the Immediate Reticular Dermis or the IRD. Once TCA has penetrated to the IRD, it becomes deeper than a medium TCA. Unfortunately, after this depth there are no further signs on the skin that can indicate the correct depth. So anything from this point onwards looks like a pure white frost. Mistakes can easily be made, and once TCA has gone too deep, it can cause irreversible damage and scarring.

Deep peels are better performed with phenol as this substance is designed to act on a deeper level of the skin and is much safer for deep peels.

There are exceptions to this rule:

There are occasions when a deeper TCA peel can be obtained for some specific conditions such as acne scarring and striae (on the body). There are two TCA variations that can do that: pixel peels and anterior chemoabrasion.

A pixel peel is a superficial TCA peel in combination with microneedling immediately before the application of the peel; this is a great treatment for acne scarring (7).

Anterior chemoabrasion is a superficial TCA peel preceded by removing part of the epidermis using a sterile fine sand paper; this is a great treatment for severe acne scarring on the face and also striae in the body (which will be explained further in Chapter 8) (8).

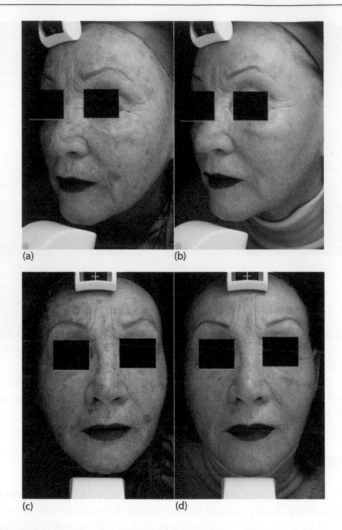

FIGURE 7.60 (a,b) Before and (c,d) after a medium-depth TCA peel of three coats.

Peeling Procedure for Pixel Peels

1) Give your patient some oral analgesia 30–45 mins before the peel.
2) Remove all makeup and cleanse the skin.
3) Cleanse the skin again with your specific pre-peel cleanser.
4) Dry the skin off.
5) Use pure alcohol to fully disinfect the skin all over with a gauze swab.
6) Then use pure acetone to fully degrease the face with a gauze swab.
7) Some practitioners prefer to do regional blocks with local anaesthesia before a pixel TCA peel. But this is generally not required.
8) Perform microneedling with either a dermaroller or dermal stamp or a dermal pen to the level of bleeding points to the full face or the area with acne scarring.
9) Take out the required amount of your TCA peel into a small dish or bowl. Do not use any formulations that contain phenol, so just stick with plain TCA products such as SkinTech Easy TCA.

10) Use one or two cotton buds to apply the TCA solution to the face. Make absolutely sure that the cotton buds are not too wet so that the TCA does not drip and run down the face or even worse in the eyes – *this is extremely dangerous.*

The face is usually divided into multiple cosmetic subunits, and the TCA is meticulously applied to the skin in an even layer. Once one area is fully covered, then move on to the next area and move around the face to complete the application in all areas.

11) Use a fan to dry the TCA on the skin and cool the face off. TCA application causes stinging and heat and can be quite uncomfortable even at low percentages.

12) There is no need to use a timer as most TCA peels are self-neutralizing and there is no need to remove them. There are, however, exceptions to this rule, so please make sure you follow the instructions according to your specific peel.

13) The expected reaction on the face is first erythema and then frosting. The desired frosting is Frosting Points or Frosting Clouds all over with a deeper white frost over the areas treated with microneedling.

14) If frosting does not appear or a deeper frosting is desired, then apply a second coat to all the areas of the face as before and dry and cool off the face with a fan.

15) Apply the recommended post-peel recovery cream and sunblock if required.

16) Give aftercare instructions to the patient.

There are many devices for microneedling available on the market (see Figure 7.61). These are automated devices that deliver microneedling at any required depth and speed. Another option for microneedling is to just use a normal hand-held dermaroller (Figure 7.62).

Figure 7.63 shows the skin being cleansed with a pre-peel cleanser. Figure 7.64 shows marking the face up according to the facial subunits (see Figure 7.21), with two extra areas that have been marked on the cheek, where acne scarring is present (Figure 7.65). These marked areas where the acne scarring is are then microneedled (Figure 7.66), resulting in erythema and pinpoint bleeding (Figure 7.67).

A 15% TCA solution is then applied to the face (Figure 7.68), including the cheeks (Figure 7.69); there is no need to apply more to the areas treated with microneedling, as the acid will automatically penetrate much deeper in these areas. Application continues to the forehead (Figure 7.70). The peel is

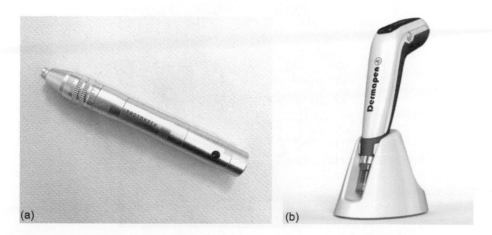

(a)   (b)

FIGURE 7.61   (a,b) Two examples of devices available on the market for microneedling.

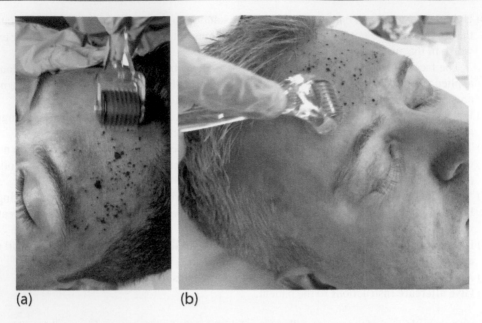

(a)   (b)

FIGURE 7.62   (a,b) Examples of microneedling with a dermaroller at 1.5mm depth. The desired outcome is pinpoint bleeding and erythema.

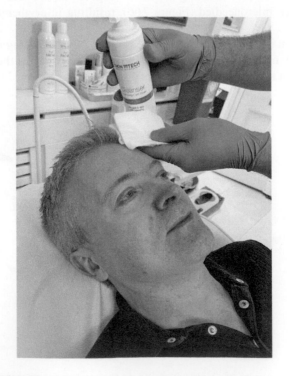

FIGURE 7.63   Cleansing the skin.

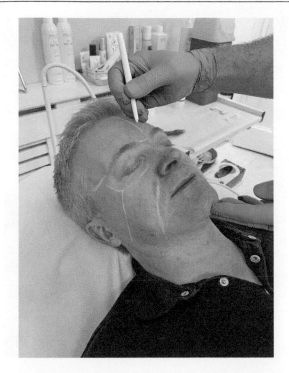

FIGURE 7.64   Marking the face into subunits.

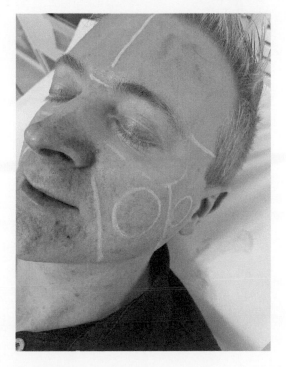

FIGURE 7.65   Additional areas marked on the cheek.

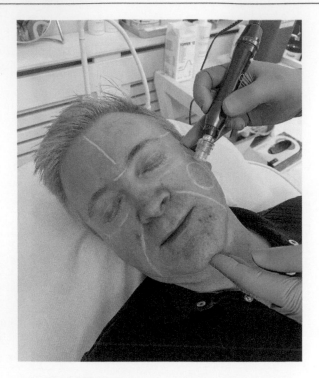

FIGURE 7.66   Microneedling the marked areas.

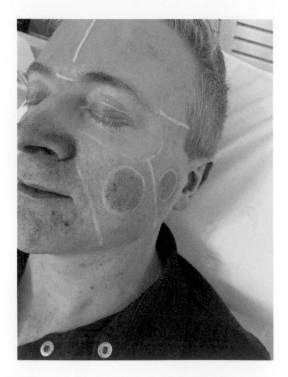

FIGURE 7.67   Erythema and pinpoint bleeding after the microneedling session.

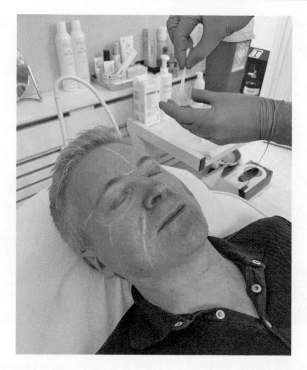

FIGURE 7.68   Applying TCA.

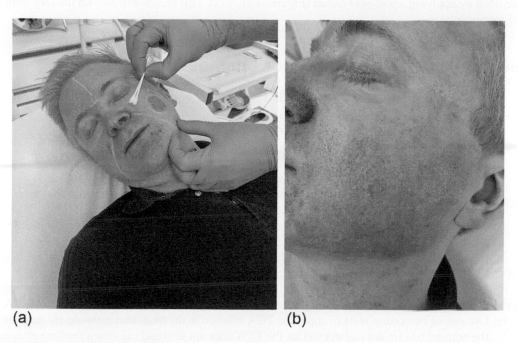

(a)   (b)

FIGURE 7.69   (a) Application to the cheeks. (b) Frosting clouds on the cheek; the frosting is more organised in the areas treated with microneedling.

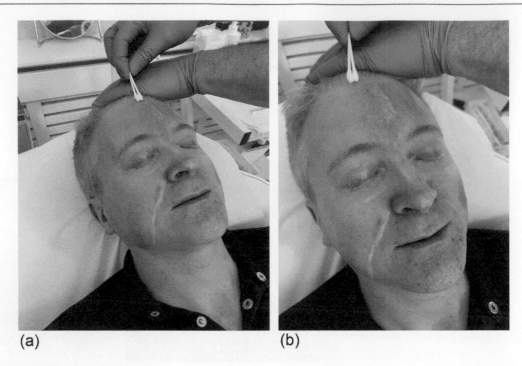

(a)   (b)

FIGURE 7.70 Applying TCA on the forehead. (a) There is already some erythema and frosting visible on the forehead; (b) A close-up of some frosting clouds on the forehead.

concluded by applying a post-peel cream (Figures 7.71, 7.72), This cream will stay on the face until the next morning.

Peeling Procedure for Anterior Chemoabrasion

1) Give your patient some oral analgesia 30–45 mins before the peel.
2) Remove all makeup and cleanse the skin.
3) Cleanse the skin again with your specific pre-peel cleanser.
4) Dry the skin off.
5) Use pure alcohol to fully disinfect the skin all over with a gauze swab.
6) Then use pure acetone to fully degrease the face with a gauze swab.
7) Some practitioners prefer to do regional blocks with local anaesthesia before an anterior chemoabrasion TCA peel.
8) Use a sterilized sandpaper which is designed for the skin and gently sand the skin down to the level of bleeding points in the area that needs treating.
9) If local anaesthesia block was not used, you can soak a gauze swab in local anaesthetic and leave it on the sanded area for 20 mins.
10) Take out the required amount of your TCA peel into a small dish or bowl. Do not use any formulations that contain phenol; just use plain TCA products such as SkinTech Easy TCA.
11) Use one or two cotton buds to apply the TCA solution to the face. Make absolutely sure that the cotton buds are not too wet so that the TCA does not drip and run down the face or even worse in the eyes – *this is extremely dangerous.*

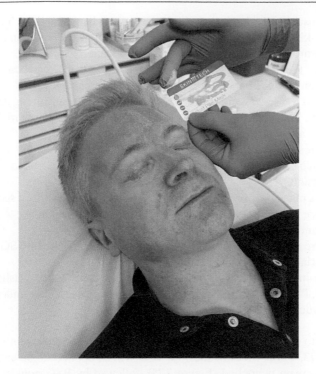

FIGURE 7.71   Applying a post-peel cream.

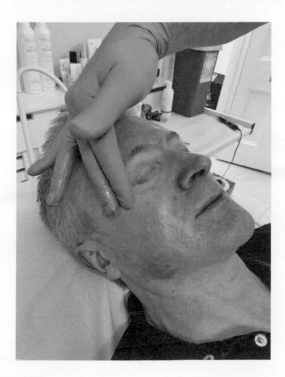

FIGURE 7.72   The end of the pixel peel procedure.

The face is usually divided into multiple cosmetic subunits, and the TCA is meticulously applied to the skin in an even layer. Once one area is fully covered, then move on to the next area and move around the face to complete the application in all areas.

12) Use a fan to dry the TCA on the skin and cool the face off. TCA application causes stinging and heat and can be quite uncomfortable even at low percentages.

13) There is no need to use a timer as most TCA peels are self-neutralizing and there is no need to remove them. There are, however, exceptions to this rule, so please make sure you follow the instructions according to your specific peel.

14) The expected reaction on the face is first erythema and then frosting. The desired frosting is frosting points or frosting clouds all over with a deeper white frost over the areas treated with sand abrasion.

15) If frosting does not appear or a deeper frosting is desired, then apply a second coat to all the areas of the face as before and dry and cool off the face with a fan.

16) Apply the recommended post-peel recovery cream.

17) Cover the entire abraded area of the face with Yellskreen powder or BSG powder. This will ensure appropriate healing of the sand-abraded areas.

18) Give aftercare instructions to the patient. The powder must not be washed off or taken off for seven days. Please refer to the section about phenol peels to fully understand how to deal with BSG powder post-peel.

The first step will be to cleanse, disinfect, and degrease the skin and then gently abrade the skin with sandpaper (Figures 7.73, 7.74). After this the 15% TCA will be applied to the entire area; frosting will appear and post-peel cream is applied (Figure 7.75), followed by BSG powder (Figure 7.76), which will have to stay in place for seven days. The result two weeks later is that there is less erythema than expected, but there is some uneven pigmentation which can be treated with tyrosinase inhibitors (Figure 7.77).

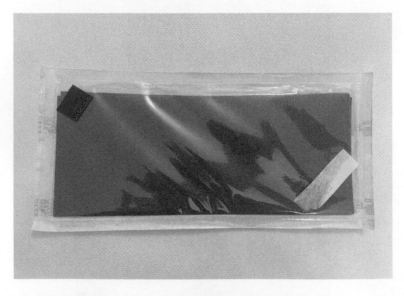

FIGURE 7.73   A pack of sterilised sandpaper for the skin used for skin abrasion.

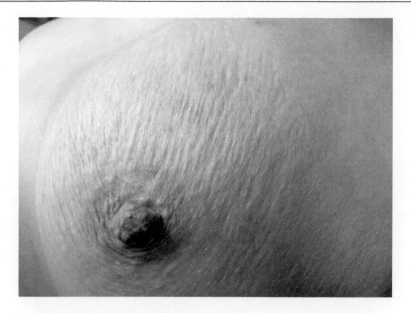

FIGURE 7.74   Breast skin with old striae after weight loss.

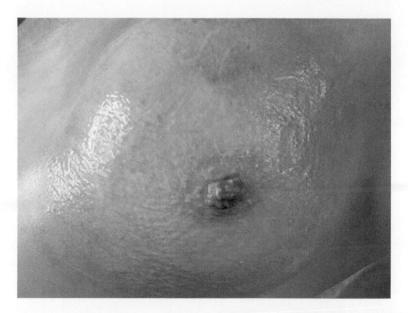

FIGURE 7.75   Breast skin with the frosting that has appeared after the peel. The post-peel cream has been applied to the area.

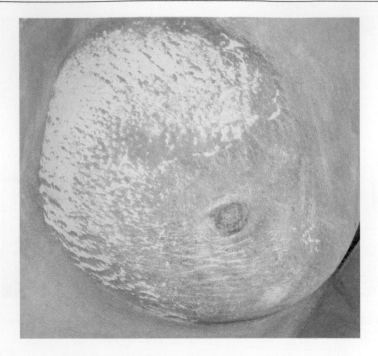

FIGURE 7.76 BSG powder has been applied to the area.

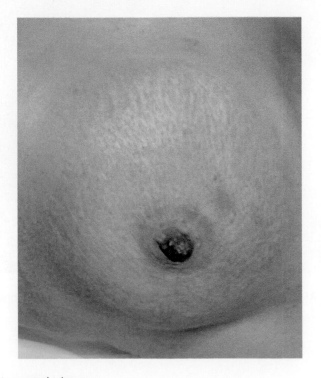

FIGURE 7.77 Result two weeks later.

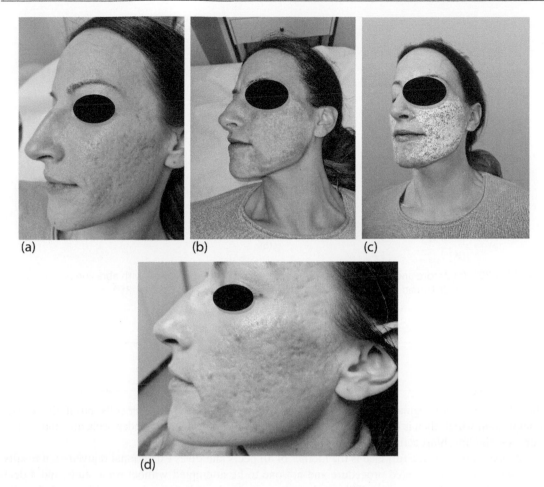

FIGURE 7.78 (a) Acne scarring on the face. (b) After a light abrasion on the acne scars, 15% TCA is applied to the face (frosting is clearly visible). (c) The next step is to cover the area in BSG powder which will have to stay on for seven days. (d) After removal of the BSG powder, about three weeks post-procedure. (Courtesy of Dr Nenad Stanković, DMD, specialist in Cosmetology, ESTERA.RS.)

Anterior chemabrasion can also be used for acne scarring on the face (Figures 7.78 and 7.79) and striae on the body (Figure 7.80).

TCA-Modified Peels

It is worth mentioning that some newer TCA-modified peels are now available on the market that allow the benefits of TCA peels without the traditional downtime of a TCA peel. These peels allow the TCA to penetrate into the dermis without epidermal damage, therefore they do not cause any frosting when applied to the skin. They cause a gradual improvement in the skin. They will help improve pigmentation and skin laxity and can be used to treat various skin conditions.

Two examples of this type of TCA peels are PhFormula and PRX-T33. For example, PRX-T33 contains 33% TCA, hydrogen peroxide (0.1-0.3%), and kojic acid 5%. This product is also very useful in the treatment of pigmentation disorders.

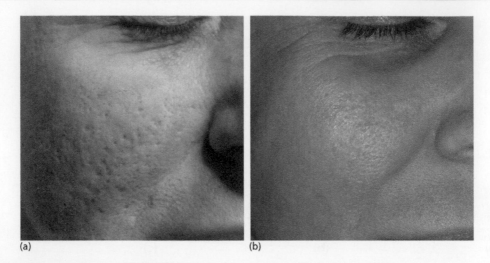

(a)　　(b)

FIGURE 7.79　(a) Before and (b) after three sessions of anterior chemabrasion with abrasion and 15% TCA peel. (Courtesy of Dr Nenad Stanković, DMD, specialist in Cosmetology, ESTERA.RS.)

PHENOL (9,10,11)

Phenol is a protein coagulating agent, so not only does it denature the living cells, but it also causes precipitation which then is defined as coagulation. It causes epidermolysis under occlusion and greatly increases the fibroblast activity in all levels of skin.

A phenol peel on the full face is the mother of all peels and gives exceptional rejuvenation results. It is, however, a complicated procedure and not one to be attempted without prior study and a deep understanding of the procedure. This peel acts on deeper levels of the dermis and goes below the immediate reticular dermis (IRD) (Figure 7.81).

At this point I should add some personal detail. It took me years to build up the knowledge and the courage to actually perform a deep phenol peel on the full face. So please take time to understand this procedure and attend as many workshops as possible to get hands-on experience or shadow someone who can teach you. I have a very busy practice in the UK, and yet to learn how to perform this peel I travelled to Paris and Barcelona multiple times; I made the time to travel a fair distance – and not just once – and I happily paid to watch the masters perform this peel. I studied their protocols and spent a few years researching the subject and studying it. So you could say that I didn't just attend a one-day course and became confident in this peel – far from it. I must mention two names here and thank them for sharing their knowledge with me on this subject, namely Dr Philip Deprez (Spain), the man behind the Lip&Eyelid Formula from SkinTech, and Dr Jean-Luc Vigneron (France), the man behind the Exopeel from Dermaceutic. Their lectures and workshops have inspired me immensely to get this far with peels.

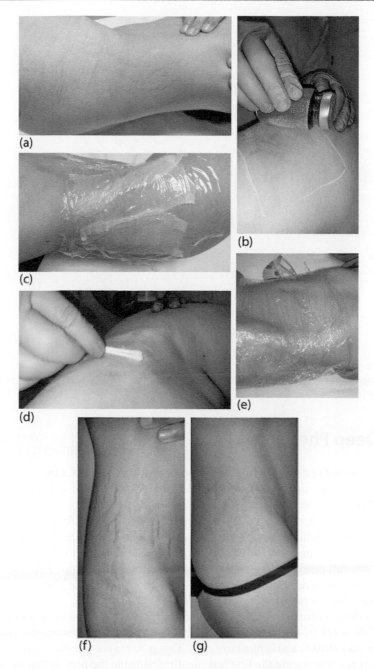

FIGURE 7.80 Anterior chemabrasion for (a) striae on the body. (b) First, the sand abrasion is completed with sandpaper; (c) lidocaine-soaked gauze swabs are then spread over the abraded area for anaesthesia. (d) The next step is to apply the 15% TCA solution. (e) After this step either one could apply BSG powder to cover the area, or in this case occlusion was been applied for 24 hours. Once the occlusion has been removed, the area will be covered with the BSG powder which will stay in place for seven days. (f and g) The final before and after pictures show an excellent result for a very difficult condition. These are the results of two treatment sessions a month apart. (Courtesy of Dr Nenad Stanković, DMD, specialist in Cosmetology, ESTERA.RS.)

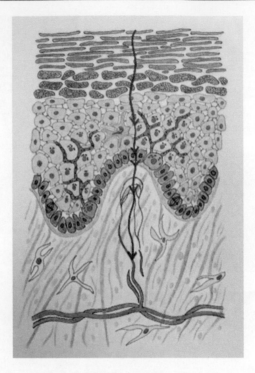

FIGURE 7.81 Phenol peel penetrates below the IRD and enters the reticular dermis to cause a deep peel with a pure white frost.

Full-Face Deep Phenol Peel

I will now explain how to perform a full-face deep phenol peel. Phenol can, of course, also only be applied to parts of the face and not necessarily to the entire face. This will be explained further in Chapter 10 (12, 13).

The process of a full-face phenol peel starts at least one month before the actual peel. The first consultation is a starting-point to looking at this peel as an option. Once the patient has expressed a positive answer, then the actual process can begin. This includes the blood test, the prescribing of the medication, and the full-face botulinum toxin treatment; I usually test for Full Blood Count (FBC), kidney and liver function (U&Es and LFTs), and if any doubt also fasting glucose and hep C serology.

The full medication list prescription can now be written out.

A full-face botulinum toxin treatment should be carried out one to two weeks before the peel. It should treat the full upper face (glabella, frontalis, and peri-orbital) and sometimes even hypermobile areas of the lower face (DAOs and orbicularis oris). This is to ensure that the expressive muscles of the face are as calm as possible during the first few months following the peel so that as many wrinkles as possible can be reduced.

Peel Day = Day Zero

It is best that the patient has not consumed a heavy breakfast just before the peel.

The patient should arrive about one hour before the procedure itself. Their hair should have been washed the night before and they should arrive without any makeup or creams on the face.

The pre-medication can now be given. It can consist of analgesia and some anxiety relief medication such as a combination of voltarol 50 mg, codeine phosphate 30 mg, and alprazolam 250 mcg.

Prepare your treatment room and treatment trolley to make sure you have everything you need at hand.

Start the procedure by gaining intravenous access with a cannula to allow administration of some IV fluids and possibly also additional analgesia. Attach 500 ml to one litre of saline or IV glucose depending on what is appropriate.

Measure the patient's blood pressure and pulse, and apply a pulse oximeter to the index finger to get constant monitoring of the oxygen saturation and the pulse. If indicated to attach a cardiac monitor, you can do so now (14).

Cover the patient with a comfortable blanket and reassure them. Cover the hair in a hair net which the patient will keep on the hair till the next morning.

Start by cleansing the face with a pre-peel cleanser, then thoroughly disinfect with alcohol and then degrease with acetone.

Then divide the face into cosmetic subunits with a white eye liner. Usually these areas are the forehead including the glabella and the upper eyelids, the cheeks including the lower eyelids, the nose, and the peri-oral area. It is best to avoid straight lines in the peri-orbital region and in the jawline to avoid obvious demarcation lines. For marking the edge of the peel near the jawline, pull the cheeks up and go under the jaw; this way the peel will include the area just below the jawline, and this will avoid obvious demarcation lines between the face and the neck.

Apply some ophthalmic ointment in the eyes.

You can decide if you want to start with the lower sections and move up or start with the forehead and move down. Let's assume we are starting with the forehead.

Inject about 2 mls of lidocaine 2% to anaesthetise both supra-orbital and supra-trochlear regions.

Take out the required amount of your phenol peel according to the manufacturer's instructions and your training and apply the first layer of the peel to the full section on the forehead. The first pass with phenol will always burn for 10–15 seconds. It is good to tell the patient you are applying the peel and count down 15 seconds to reassure them. After 15 seconds the burning sensation will disappear. Make sure you take about five minutes to apply the phenol to the entire area by going over the area and allowing the oil-based solution to penetrate the skin. Depending on the thickness or the oiliness of the skin and how well the skin was prepared, you may or may not see a full white frost. Often you will see immediate erythema and some oedema. You can apply two to three layers of the peel to the forehead. Subsequent layers will not burn at all. It is likely that you will then see a full white frost on the whole section.

Once the forehead is finished, move on to the upper eyelids. (I sometimes choose to peel the entire face and finish with the eyelids at the end. It doesn't really matter.) Take the required amount of peel for the eyelid. Soak a single small cotton bud with the peel solution. Make absolutely sure it is not dripping wet.

Apply the first coat of the peel to the upper eyelid, but avoiding the upper lid tarsus. Again help the patient cope with the burning by counting down the 15 seconds. You should see an immediate full white frost. Apply the second coat; this will no longer burn. Repeat on the other upper eyelid.

Now we have to wait around 10–15 minutes before we move to the next area. This rest period between sections allows the phenol to be metabolised and is a good safety measure. We can use this rest period to apply the occlusive tape to the forehead section, or if not needed apply the after-peel cream and the BSG powder. The application of the tape takes some time. The tape has to be cut into small sections with sterile scissors and meticulously applied to the whole area to make sure it stays in full contact with the whole skin for 24 hours. The upper edge of the tapes near the hairline can be overlaid with some gauze swabs overlapping the hairnet. More occlusive tape can be used to attach the upper section of the forehead to the gauze swab and the hairnet. This will make it much easier to take the tape off the next day by just pulling it down with the hairnet.

I would then usually move on to the nose and apply two to three layers to the entire nose, including the ala and the columella and the glabella, on the same principles as above. Then use the rest period to either cover with the tape or just cream and BSG. If applying the tape, you will have to cut the tape into very small sections to be able to cover the entire nose.

The next area is the cheeks and lower eyelids. Apply lidocaine 2% to cover the infra-orbital region. It is also helpful to apply some local anaesthetic to the pre-auricular region and alongside the jawline. The cheeks and the lower eyelids do not need any more than two coats of the peel generally. Again apply the peel taking your time to ensure a good reaction on the whole section. When applying the peel to the lower eyelids, only use one cotton bud ensuring it is not dripping wet. Pull the eyelid down near the cheek-lid junction and ask the patient to keep looking up. Apply the peel as close as you can to about 2mm away from the lash line. The first pass will give a perfect full white frost. Apply a second layer and then put more ophthalmic ointment in the eye.

Again use the 15-minute rest period to cover this area with tape or the BSG powder.

After 15 minutes repeat the process on the other cheek and lower eyelid and use the rest period to cover it up.

The final area is the peri-oral area. Apply a mental nerve block with lidocaine 2%, and if necessary apply more infra-orbital infiltration to ensure the upper lip is anaesthetised. The peri-oral area typically needs three coats of the peel solution. It is best to apply a little bit of the peel into the individual wrinkles first to ensure full frosting of the base of each wrinkle before applying it to the full area.

You can apply the peel into the red area of the lip just next to the vermillion border. This will ensure full removal of all peri-oral lines.

Finally, cover this last area with the occlusive tapes or the BSG powder.

This is officially the end of the peel. Feel free to give more analgesia if needed. At this stage most patients feel some throbbing of the face. I find that some IV Toradol actually helps, and they obviously have their paracetamol-codeine pain relief to take at the hotel.

It is best to keep the patient in the clinic for maybe 30–60 minutes and to offer them a drink with a straw and any oral analgesia (and, of course, their next dose of acyclovir).

Most patients are relatively comfortable at this stage. My advice is always to go home and get into bed. Take your pain relief; take another alprazolam and try and sleep it off. The pain will stop. Preparing the patient for this and reassuring them always helps them to get through it. After this initial period of pain due to inflammation, the pain will completely stop and the rest of the recovery process is completely pain-free.

Once they go back to their house or hotel room, it is *very* important that they sleep with a few pillows behind their back, to stay slightly upright, with a fan cooling off the face continuously. I find cooling off the face will help tremendously with the post-peel pain which will kick in and last for four to eight hours.

Figure 7.82a shows the typical equipment required for a phenol peel – in this case, a SkinTech phenol peel – some gloves, a container for the acid, some cotton buds, a pre-peel cleanser, gauze swabs, some ophthalmic ointment, post-peel cream, alcohol, acetone, and some BSG powder. Figure 7.82b shows the equipment for a full-face phenol peel with occlusion – a 60% phenol kit from SkinTech called Lip&Eyelid formula, scissors, gauze swabs, dispensing dish, needles, and syringes of various sizes. Figure 7.82c shows shows more equipment being prepared – pre-peel cleansers, alcohol, acetone, a marking pencil, ophthalmic ointment, needles and syringes, a pulse oximeter, and a small portable ECG checker. We will also need a blood pressure monitor and an ECG monitor to attach to the patient.

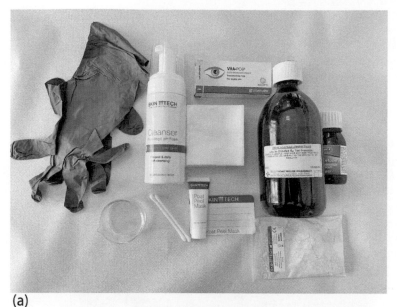

(a)

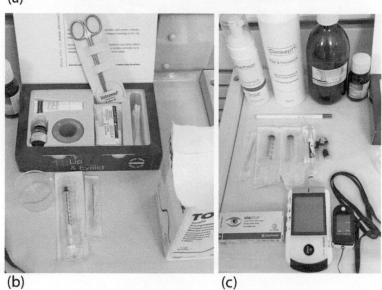

(b)   (c)

FIGURE 7.82   (a) Equipment for a phenol peel; (b) equipment for a full-face phenol peel with occlusion; (c) further equipment.

An IV line will need to be established with saline, and all the pre-medication will need to be given to the patient about half an hour or so before the procedure.

Figure 7.83 shows cleansing the face and then disinfecting it fully with alcohol; Figure 7.84 shows use of acetone to degrease the face completely. Figure 7.85 shows marking up the different zones of the face and also the areas to be injected to obtain a facial block per area, as I move through the various sections. Ophthalmic ointment is then applied to the eyes before the procedure (Figure 7.86). I then do an infra-orbital block using lidocaine (Figure 7.87), as I will be starting with the lower face and moving up. If I had decided to start with the forehead, I would have done a supra-orbital and supra-trochlear block first.

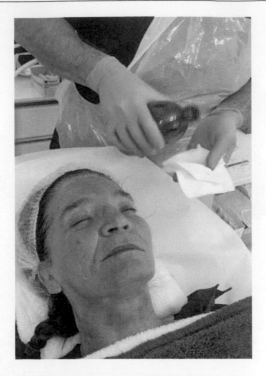

FIGURE 7.83   Cleansing the face and disinfecting it with alcohol.

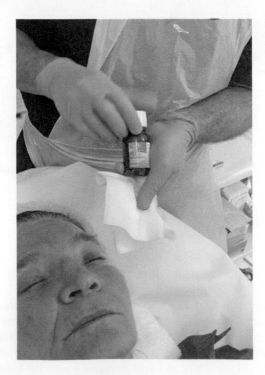

FIGURE 7.84   Using acetone to degrease the face.

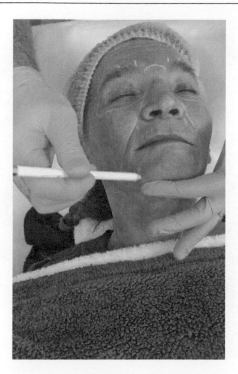

FIGURE 7.85   Marking up different zones of the face.

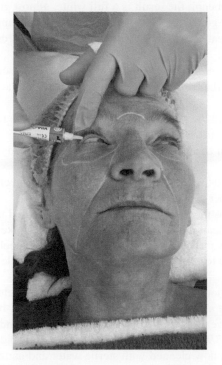

FIGURE 7.86   Applying ophthalmic ointment.

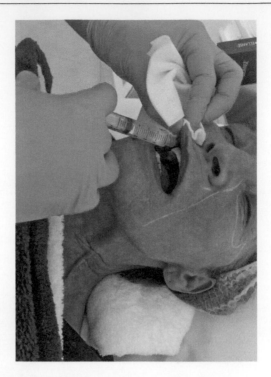

FIGURE 7.87   An infra-orbital block using lidocaine.

I treat the top with 60% phenol; the result is a full white, almost grey-looking frost (Figure 7.88). This means we have definitely gone below the IRD. The peel is then applied on the lower lip and chin area after a mental block application with lidocaine; again the desired result is a full white frost (Figure 7.89).

The nose is then treated; a nice deep frost should form on the nose, and the top lip and chin areas should 'defrost', which means the frost is disappearing and being replaced with erythema and oedema (Figure 7.90).

Occlusive tape is applied to the nose, top lip, and chin during the rest period, and the peel is then applied on the cheek area (Figure 7.91).

The lower eyelids are then treated; the cheeks should have already almost completely 'defrosted' by now (Figure 7.92).

Occlusive tape is applied to the cheeks; more ophthalmic solution can be placed in the eyes and the peel is then applied on the upper eyelid (Figure 7.93).

The peel is now applied to the last area of the face being treated now, namely the forehead. The supra-orbital and supra-trochlear block with lidocaine help to make everything very comfortable (Figure 7.94). Occlusive tape is placed on the forehead to finish the peel (Figures 7.95 and 7.96).

The patient will now need to try and be very still during the whole night so that the tape does not come off.

Figure 7.97 shows the patient the morning after her peel: the occlusive tape is still fully in place and there should be no pain at all. It is to be expected that there will be a lot of peri-orbital oedema. The mask is now removed, revealing the skin; the occlusive mask tends to come off in one go and is not painful to remove (Figure 7.98). The skin tends to look wet and epidermal liquefaction may be evident (Figure 7.99). The face is now cleaned with sterile water and gauze swabs, and a post-peel mask is applied (Figure 7.100). BSG powder is applied to the entire face (Figure 7.101); this powder must not

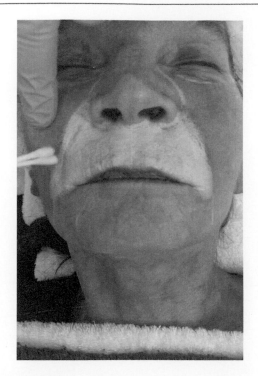

FIGURE 7.88   Top lip treated with phenol.

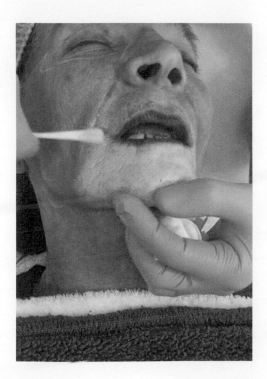

FIGURE 7.89   Treating lower lip and chin.

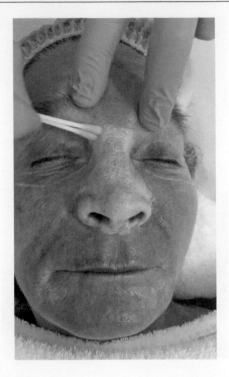

FIGURE 7.90 Treating the nose.

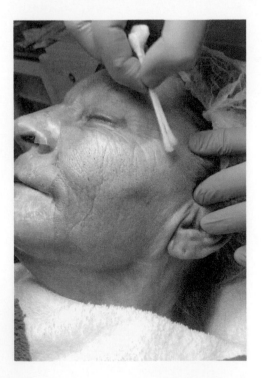

FIGURE 7.91 Treating the cheek area.

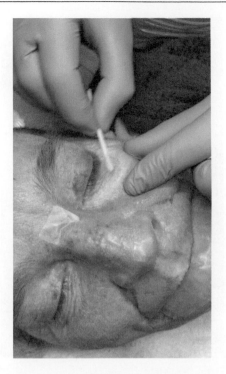

FIGURE 7.92   Treating the lower eyelids, with a pure white frost forming.

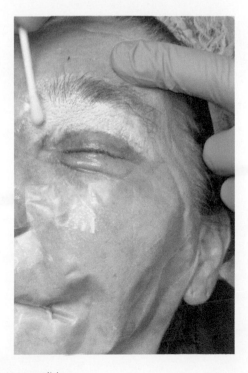

FIGURE 7.93   Treating the upper eyelid.

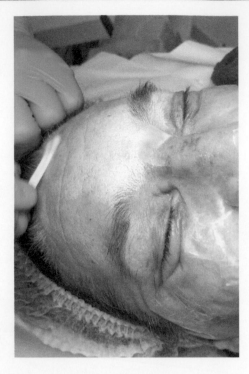

FIGURE 7.94   Treating the forehead; a pure white frost is forming in this area.

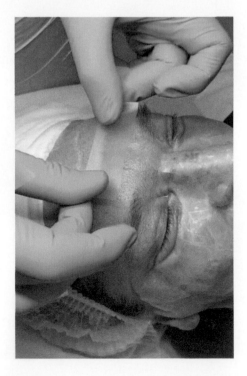

FIGURE 7.95   Applying occlusive tape.

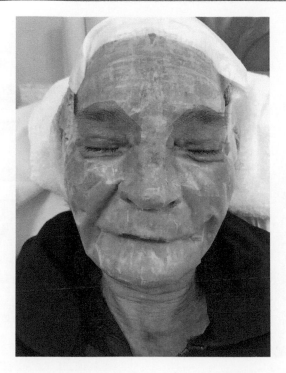

FIGURE 7.96 Immediately after the procedure.

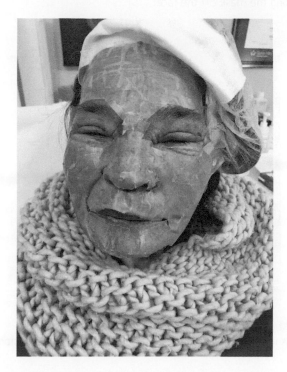

FIGURE 7.97 The morning after the peel (i.e., day one of the peel).

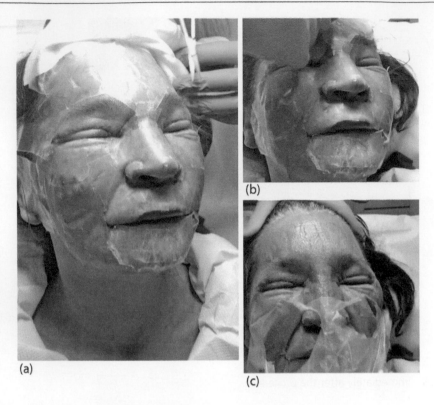

FIGURE 7.98 (a,b,c) Taking the mask off the face.

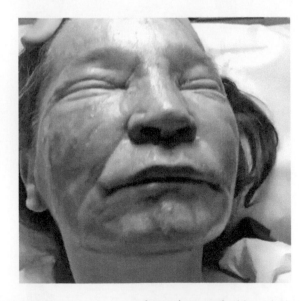

FIGURE 7.99 The skin as it appears on day one after a deep peel with occlusion.

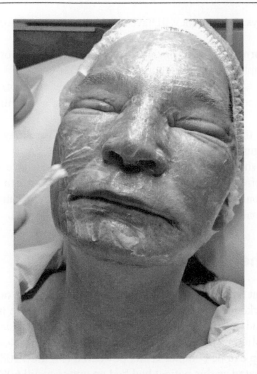

FIGURE 7.100   Applying the post-peel mask on the face.

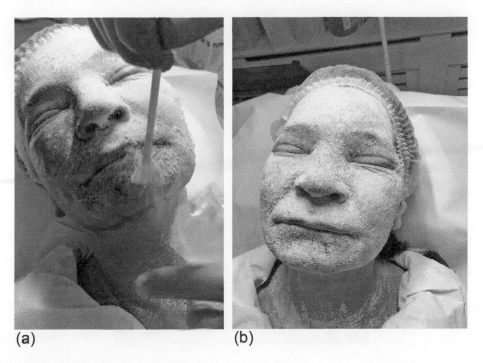

(a)   (b)

FIGURE 7.101   (a,b) Applying BSG powder onto the entire face.

get washed off for seven days. The patient will have to take extra powder home to keep applying powder in areas that become wet.

The patient should return to the clinic on day three for review; more powder should be applied even if there are no signs of complications or infection (Figure 7.102).

By day seven some parts of the BSG crust may have already come off (Figure 7.103). The patient will have to apply an ointment to the entire face overnight so that everything can come off the following morning.

By six months most of the wrinkles should have vanished. There may be some residual erythema which will settle down (Figure 7.104).

By one year the face should look great. The erythema should have completely gone and there should be a great visible correction of most of the ageing signs. It is worth mentioning that the patient shown in Figure 7.105 had only this one peel treatment and no further treatments were carried out after the peel during these 12 months, so any noticeable effect is from the peel.

Full-Face Light Phenol Peel

Figure 7.106 shows a patient ready to receive a light phenol peel at 30% on the full face, having been cleansed, prepped, and marked up. Phenol is applied to the forehead, the nose, and the right cheek in turn, with a pause of around 15 minutes in between the areas. If occlusion is not being applied, the BSG powder can been applied to the areas that have so far been completed (Figure 7.107). The left cheek and then the upper lip can be completed and powdered (Figure 7.108). The upper eyelids shown in Figure 7.109 were not treated as this patient had had an upper eyelid 60% phenol peel (mosaic peel) a few years ago.

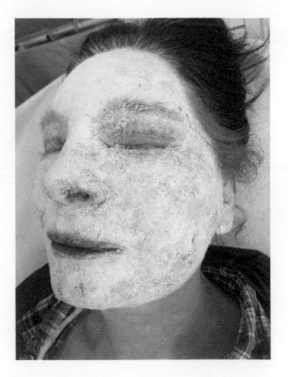

FIGURE 7.102   Patient on day three (in clinic).

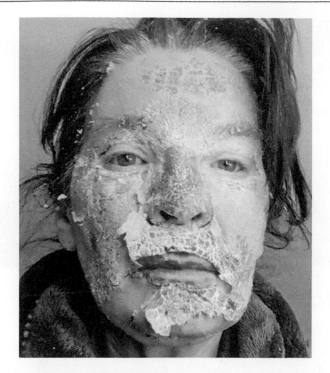

FIGURE 7.103   Patient in day seven (at home).

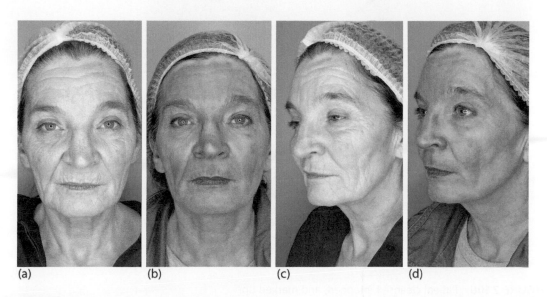

(a)   (b)   (c)   (d)

FIGURE 7.104   (a, c) Before and (b, d) six months after.

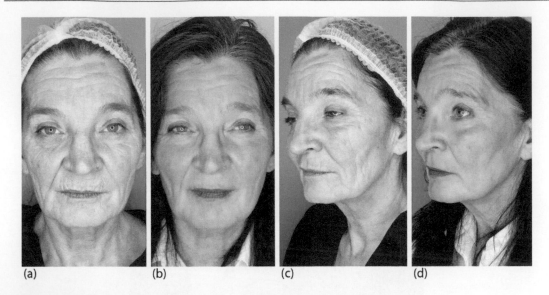

(a)　　　　　(b)　　　　　(c)　　　　　(d)

FIGURE 7.105　(a, c) Before and (b, d) one year after.

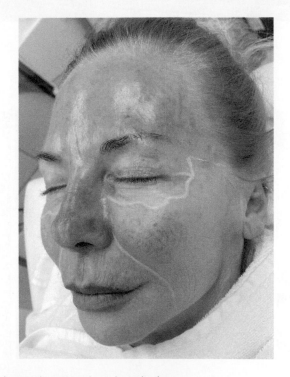

FIGURE 7.106　Patient cleansed, prepped, and marked up.

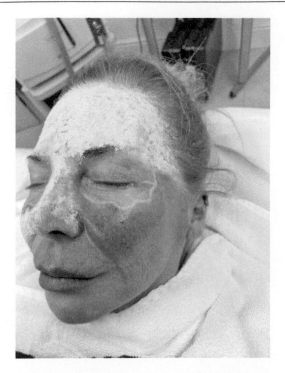

FIGURE 7.107 Treatment completed for the forehead, nose, and right cheek.

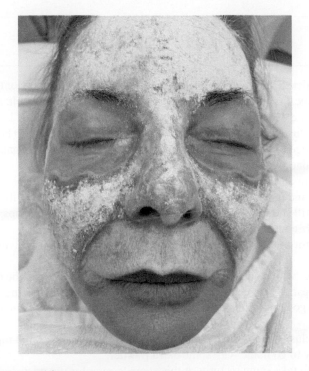

FIGURE 7.108 Treatment completed for the left cheek.

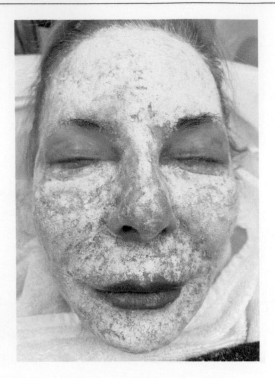

FIGURE 7.109   Treatment of the full face except for the upper eyelids.

DAY ONE REVIEW (15)

This is a relatively quick review which takes between 15 and 30 minutes only. Usually the patient comes back to the clinic first thing in the morning. At this stage most people are unable to properly open their eyes due to the oedema; they are guided to the treatment room.

If the adhesive occlusive tapes were applied to the face, they will need to be taken off first.

Grasp the upper edge of the adhesive tape layer that was attached to the gauze swabs, and pull the mask off rapidly with one swift movement; this is generally not painful.

Clean the face from any exudate with sterile swabs and saline.

Have a good look and make sure that all wrinkles have 'disappeared', as the epidermis has macerated. If any wrinkles still show, now is the time to perform very small touch-ups with the same product just into the base of those wrinkles.

Then cover the entire face with the after-peel cream and then start applying the BSG powder to the full face.

Clean the eyelashes with some wet cotton buds and see if you can open the eyes with your fingers. Often this allows the patient to see a little bit; feel free to put some hydrating eye drops in the eyes. The patient is ready to go home with some extra BSG powder to re-apply when necessary over the next couple of days.

If no adhesive occlusive tapes were applied, then just clean the eyes and top up the BSG powder, and the patient is ready to go home with some extra powder.

It is always good to take some pictures at this stage to monitor progress.

DAY THREE REVIEW

This review is usually no longer than 15 minutes, and it is to ensure that the patient is not developing any sign of infection. This is usually noticeable as a red rash on the neck or below the jawline. It is very rare for this to happen, especially when prophylactic antibiotics are given. Feel free to touch up the BSG powder if necessary, and if any visible dry cracks near the mouth corners, near the eyes, or the jawline, feel free to add a small amount of Fucidin ointment with a small cottonbud.

For patients who live far away this tends to be a virtual visit.

TWO-WEEK REVIEW

During this review the state of the new skin is assessed to ensure there are no issues with the healing process. It is normal to have a lot of erythema at this point, but any areas of delayed healing should ring alarm bells and need to be monitored carefully to avoid scarring. At this stage most patients are loving their new skin and are using their aftercare products; some also use makeup to cover up the erythema (Figure 7.110).

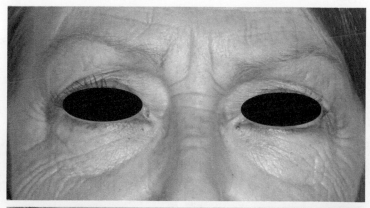
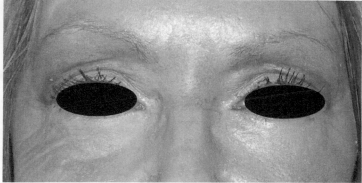

FIGURE 7.110   Before and two weeks after pictures of a patient who had a phenol peel on the entire face including the eyelids. The face was treated with a 30% phenol formula while the eyelids received 60% phenol. The level of skin tightening is already very noticeable. Patient is wearing makeup to hide the erythema.

It is important to mention to the patient that minor peeling may happen for another week or two as the skin adjusts itself. Also worth mentioning is that as the oedema settles, some areas may gain look a bit deflated, but they will improve again in a few months' time as the neocollagenesis kicks in.

THREE-MONTH REVIEW

At this stage most patients have got the full effect of the peel and are very happy. In some cases erythema may still persist a little bit.

Check the skin at this stage for any milia that may need to be removed with the tip of a needle, and also consider some IPL or laser treatment for any telangiectasia that the patient may wish to remove.

SIX-MONTH REVIEW

After six months the final full results are visible and the official after pictures can now be taken (Figures 7.111 to 7.114).

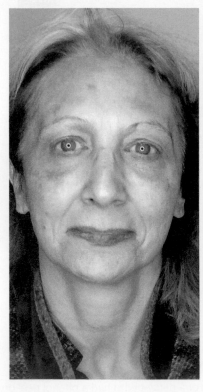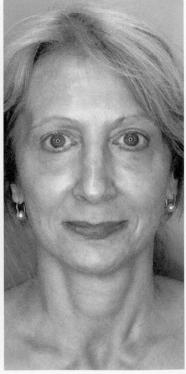

FIGURE 7.111   Results about six months after a 60% phenol peel on the full face to treat skin laxity and pigmentation.

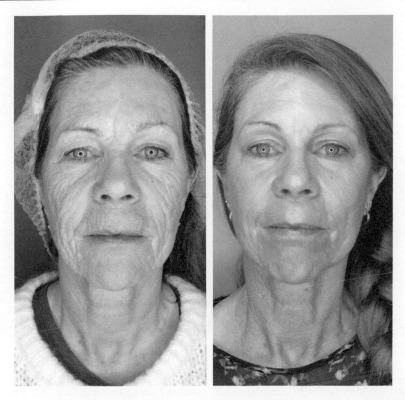

FIGURE 7.112   Results about six months after a 60% phenol peel with full-face occlusion to treat solar elastosis.

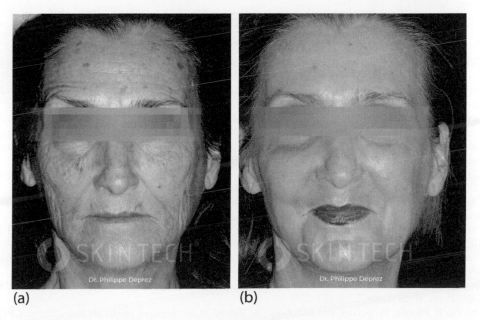

(a)   (b)

FIGURE 7.113   (a) Before and (b) after photographs of a full-face 60% phenol peel with full-face occlusion (using Lip&Eyelid Formula SkinTech). (Courtesy of Dr Philippe Deprez PhD and Skin Tech Pharma Group.)

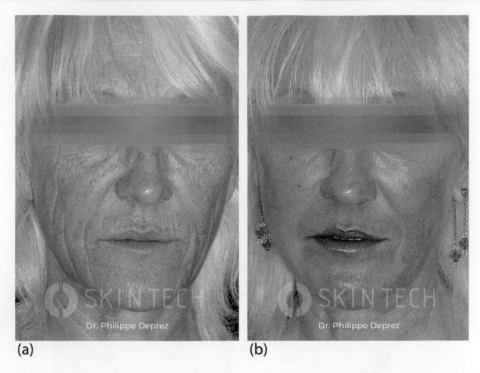

(a)   (b)

FIGURE 7.114   (a) Before and (b) after photographs of a full-face 60% phenol peel with full-face occlusion (using Lip&Eyelid Formula SkinTech). (Courtesy of Dr Philippe Deprez PhD and Skin Tech Pharma Group.)

REFERENCES

1. Deprez P, Alpha hydroxy acids: Chemistry, pH and pKa, and mechanism of action, in: *Textbook of chemical peels*, second edition, CRC Press, Boca Raton, 2016: 45–47.
2. Deprez P, Trichloracetic acid: General information, toxicity, formulations and histology, in: *Textbook of chemical peels*, second edition, CRC Press, Boca Raton, 2016: 74–88.
3. Obagi ZE, Overview of TCA and other chemical peels, in: *Skin health restoration and rejuvenation*, Springer, New York, 2000: 112–126.
4. Deprez P, Trichloracetic acid: Classic semiology, in: *Textbook of chemical peels*, second edition, CRC Press, Boca Raton, 2016: 98–101.
5. Obagi ZE, The blue peel, endpoints, in: *Skin health restoration and rejuvenation*, Springer, New York, 2000: 165–172.
6. Obagi ZE, The Obagi controlled medium-depth peel, significance of endpoints, in: *Skin health restoration and rejuvenation*, Springer, New York, 2000: 204–211.
7. Deprez P, Combination peels, microneedling pixel peel, in: *Textbook of chemical peels*, second edition, CRC Press, Boca Raton, 2016: 380–382.
8. Deprez P, Stretch marks, scars and pilar keratosis: Anterior chemabrasion, in: *Textbook of chemical peels second edition*, CRC Press, Boca Raton, 2016: 152–182.
9. Deprez P, Phenol: Chemistry, formulations and adjuvants, in: *Textbook of chemical peels*, second edition, CRC Press, Boca Raton, 2016: 211–220.
10. Deprez P, Phenol: Properties and histology, in: *Textbook of chemical peels*, second edition: CRC Press, Boca Raton, 2016: 221–225.

11. Deprez P, Phenol: Indications, in: *Textbook of chemical peels*, second edition, CRC Press, Boca Raton: 250–263.
12. Deprez P, Full-face phenol: Nerve block anesthesia and/or sedation, in: *Textbook of chemical peels*, second edition, CRC Press, Boca Raton, 2016: 275–284.
13. Deprez P, Full-face phenol: Application, in: *Textbook of chemical peels*, second edition, CRC Press, Boca Raton, 2016: 285–294.
14. Deprez P, Phenol toxicity: Causes, prevention and treatment, in: *Textbook of chemical peels*, second edition, CRC Press, Boca Raton, 2016: 230–238.
15. Deprez P, Full-face phenol: Postpeel care, in: *Textbook of chemical peels*, second edition, CRC Press, Boca Raton, 2016: 295–306.

Body Procedures

8

Any body area can be treated with a chemical peel. The biggest rule to remember is that the skin on the body has far less density of pilosebaceous units and is therefore slower when it comes to healing; body areas generally take twice as long to heal. So if, say, the time off after a face peel is one week, you should make that two weeks for any body parts. Deep peels are contra-indicated on the body, as they would lead to scarring. The only way to get around this issue is to perform an anterior chemoabrasion, which will be explained in this chapter.

I am now going to discuss the most common areas of the body treated with peels, namely the neck and decolletage, the back of the hands, and the striae.

NECK AND DECOLLETAGE (1)

Once patients see the improvement on their face, they can start looking elsewhere, and for many female patients the first area that they notice is the neck and the decolletage. The most common problem here is skin laxity, thin skin, wrinkles, and sun damage. Superficial peels are great for this area but will need a course of treatment.

The best peel for this area is a peel to the Grenz zone with TCA. One is looking to achieve a good level of frosting clouds all over the entire area. Medium TCA peels are possible in this area in people with very thick skin, but you still need to be very cautious; remember there is more risk of scarring in this area compared to the face, so we are not looking to get full white frosting here.

Again, the procedure starts with a consultation where options are explained to the patient about various available treatments for this area. Peels can, of course, be combined with many other treatments such as lasers, IPL, radiofrequency, ultherapy, BodyTite, mesotherapy, PRP, etc. – not, of course, all at the same time but as part of a treatment protocol combining various treatments. Always remember that a course of treatment is necessary to get optimum results.

The next thing is skin preparation. Just like the face, the skin on the neck and decolletage can be prepared with products. The same rules apply. Most women already use their face products on their neck and decolletage anyway, but sunscreen is the only product that is often forgotten in this area, so again reminding your patient about the importance of sun protection is always very important.

As the skin takes longer to heal, the healing phase products will need to be used for longer and the desquamation will be delayed compared to the face.

The neck and decolletage can of course be peeled at the same time as the face; however, remember that more product may be needed to cover all areas for the treatment.

Figure 8.1 shows the desquamation after a TCA peel on the back of the neck. Due to a good level of thickness of the skin in this area, the peel was nearly at medium depth, hence the pronounced large scales of dry skin coming off around day five.

Figure 8.2 shows the skin immediately after two coats of 15% TCA application on the neck and decolletage. We can clearly see erythema and plenty of frosting clouds.

DOI: 10.1201/9781003244134-8

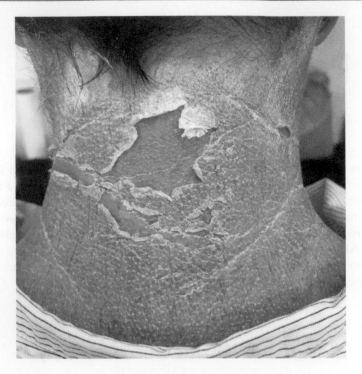

FIGURE 8.1 Desquamation after a TCA peel on the back of the neck.

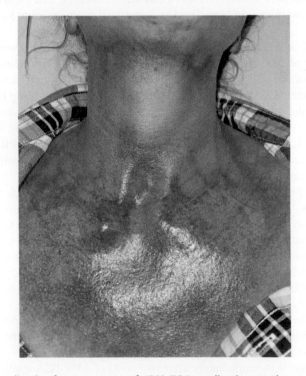

FIGURE 8.2 Skin immediately after two coats of 15% TCA application on the neck and decolletage.

BACK OF THE HANDS (2,3)

This is a real 'give away' area. Often it is the back of the hand that tells the real age of the patient and not necessarily their face. Problems in this area are usually loss of skin elasticity, sun damage, lentigines, and loss of subcutaneous volume; the loss of volume is usually treated successfully with a plethora of filling agents. The results are usually very good.

The skin itself can benefit enormously from a course of peels. I would again recommend TCA peels for this area. Only superficial peels to the basal layer or Grenz zone are recommended here. Medium TCA peels are best avoided.

You could discuss treatment options for this area during a consultation. Often patients do not come to us to treat their hands. They come to treat their face. However, after the face has been treated, then perhaps we should mention to them that we can also help them to get younger-looking hands. Trust me – even patients who have been coming to me for many years for their face sometimes forget that their hands are ageing as well. So a gentle reminder or a leaflet to take away is always a good idea and will lead to follow-up treatments.

For the hands, a bit like the neck area, discuss various treatment options that may be combined as part of a treatment protocol.

Skin preparation for the hands is generally not necessary but again using AHA-based products or some form of retinoid will of course enhance the results. The most important thing is not to forget sun protection for this area as well. Due to constant washing of hands it is hard to keep the hands protected all day long. So it might be a good idea to carry a small tube of sunscreen in the handbag all day and use it as a hand cream.

Remember to have at least two weeks between peels in this area to allow full recovery of the skin.

How do we remove lentigines from the back of the hands? The best solution for this is to use a focal deep TCA peel, which we discussed earlier on. A great example of such a peel is SkinTech Only Touch. This is a 45% TCA peel, which should *never* be applied to large areas – in fact, no larger than 5mm in diameter! This peel needs to be applied very carefully to the lentigo itself with a very fine cotton bud. One or two touches are generally enough to get a full white frost over the lentigo. Once the frosting has appeared on the lentigo (lentigines), then follow with a superficial TCA like SkinTech Easy TCA to the entire area of the back of the hand, including the already-treated lentigines.

This specific protocol recommends a course of four TCA peels where the first and the fourth peel are combined with Only Touch. Each peel is performed every 15 days. Again, other products and other manufacturers will have their own specific protocols, so please make sure you always follow the protocol you have been taught with your own specific range of products.

The results of such treatment are very successful and long-lasting. When combined with volume replacement, this really completely rejuvenates the hands to match the face.

Figure 8.3 shows the hands of a patient with multiple lentigines before any treatment.

Figure 8.4 shows preparation for treatment. The hands have been cleansed. In the left receptacle I have a small amount of 45% TCA with a small applicator, and on the right receptacle I have a 15% TCA and cotton buds for the application.

Figure 8.5 shows application of the 45% TCA to the individual lentigines. Care has to be taken to treat the entire lentigo and to go just slightly outside of its borders so that no remnant pigment is left around the treated area.

Figure 8.6 shows the hands after the application of the 45% TCA to all the lentigines. This deep focal TCA application cause white-grey frosting indicating that the acid has penetrated below the IRD. At this stage, one or two coats of 15% TCA will be applied to the entire back of the hands to even out the peel.

Figure 8.7 shows the patient one week post-procedure. It is quite normal for the deep focally treated areas to scab over. It will take at least two to three weeks until full recovery.

Figure 8.8 shows the result after three weeks. The lentigines have gone, but there are still some areas of erythema where the deeper TCA was focally applied. This erythema will settle down over the next few weeks.

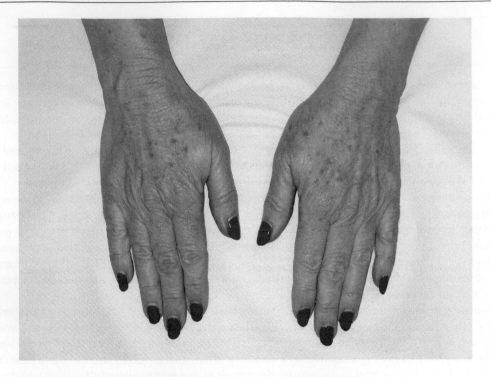

FIGURE 8.3   Multiple lentigines before any treatment.

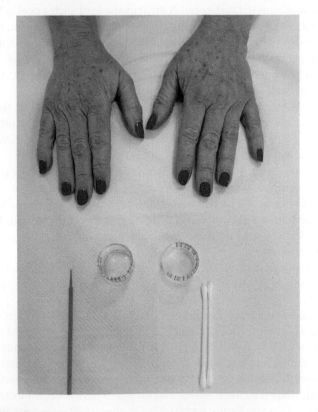

FIGURE 8.4   Preparation for treatment.

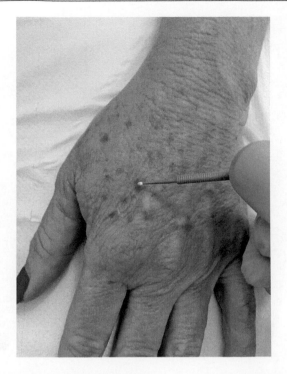

FIGURE 8.5   Application of TCA to individual lentigines.

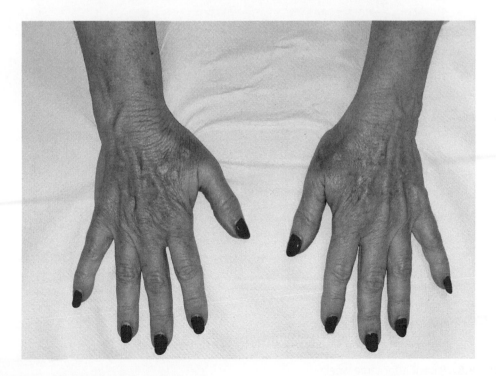

FIGURE 8.6   After application.

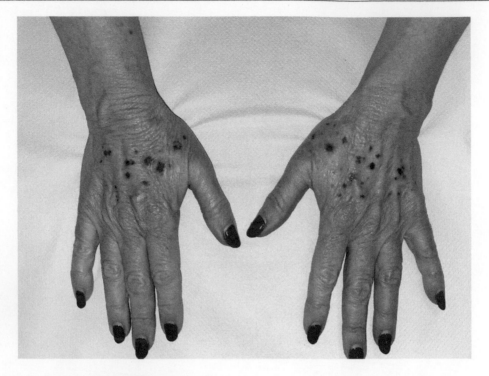

FIGURE 8.7   Patient after one week.

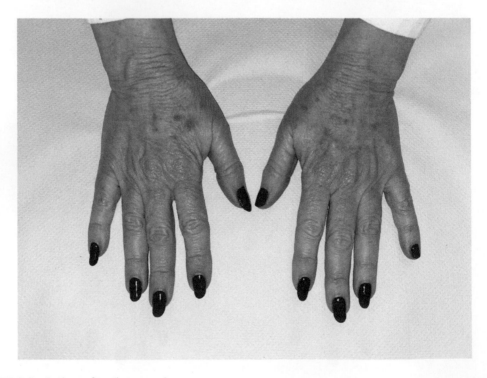

FIGURE 8.8   Patient after three weeks.

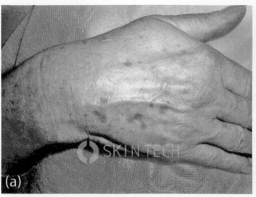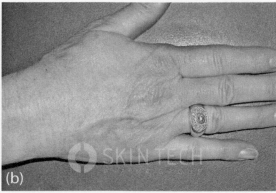

FIGURE 8.9 (a) Before and (b) after results of a complete procedure using focal 45% TCA (Only Touch SkinTech) and 15% TCA (Easy TCA SkinTech). (Courtesy of Dr Philippe Deprez, PhD, Skin Tech Pharma Group.)

Figure 8.9 shows the before and after results of a complete procedure using focal 45% TCA (Only Touch SkinTech) and 15% TCA (Easy TCA SkinTech).

STRIAE (4)

Striae, or stretch marks, are not easy to treat; everybody knows that. Various types of light-based devices can be used – microneedling, dermarollers, PRP, mesotherapy, pixel peels, etc. When striae are fresh and red, lasers are very useful. However, in old white striae this becomes harder.

A treatment that is fairly successful for this condition is anterior chemoabrasion (AC) with occlusion. An AC can allow deep penetration of a superficial peel in areas where deep peelings are contraindicated. It has a superior rejuvenating and repairing effect on striae, compared to – for example – a pixel peel. However, this is a very specific protocol, so please make sure you have had adequate training for this procedure before trying it.

Start with the skin preparation. Retinoids are in my opinion very useful in preparation for the treatment of striae or any type of scarring. I would recommend once or even twice daily use of tretinoin, perhaps mixed with hydroquinone 4% to allow better penetration of the tretinoin and also to prep the skin to avoid PIH. PIH can be common with this procedure, so prepare well and treat afterwards with the same combination of tretinoin and hydroquinone. Prepare the skin for at least a couple of weeks. Always remember to stop the use of retinoids and/or hydroquinone a good week before any actual peeling procedure.

The protocol starts by using a very fine-grade sterilized skin sandpaper (which you can get from SkinTech, for example). Use the sandpaper gently on the surface of the skin and cover the entire area with the striae. There is no analgesia necessary. If you are causing pain, you have gone too deep. We are looking to remove part of the epidermis and to expose a small percentage of the very tips of the dermal papillae. So you should see very small pin-prick blood points when doing this. Once this has been completed, gauze swabs soaked in local anaesthetic are placed on the skin and left in place to create some local anaesthesia.

After this, a normal superficial TCA peel is performed – for example – EasyTCA (15% TCA). After the peel the after-peel cream is applied and then immediately the area is covered with cling film for 24 hours.

This is the only protocol where I have seen occlusion being applied after a TCA peel. This protocol is not suitable for the face.

The patient goes home, keeping the area completely covered with cling film overnight. They will return the next day and the cling film is removed. It is normal to have exudate accumulating under the plastic; this needs to be cleaned with sterile gauze swabs and some sterile saline.

At this stage the skin is extremely erythematous and possibly swollen. The treated section of the skin will now need to be covered with BSG powder (the same powder used after a phenol peel).

Just like a phenol peel, the BSG must not be washed off for at least seven days. Once the skin has healed, the scabs and the rest of the BSG can be removed by applying a thick ointment to the area overnight to let it soak (just like a phenol peel on the face).

The post-peel erythema will need to be treated with your aftercare products and sun protection if the area is exposed to daylight.

Any PIH will need to be treated with anti-oxidants, anti-tyrosinase products, and sunscreen as usual.

Figure 8.10 shows a typical example of striae on the abdomen, which can be extremely difficult to get rid of. Sometimes a combination of treatments will be necessary to improve this condition.

Figure 8.11 shows treatment of a breast covered in old striae after weight loss; the result is shown after one session of AC. The uneven skin colour will be treated with tyrosinase inhibitors to blend everything in.

Figure 8.12 shows the result of an AC treatment with occlusion on striae on the body; two treatments were performed a month apart.

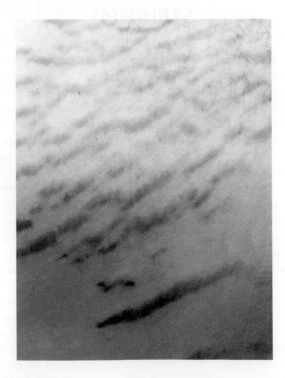

FIGURE 8.10 Striae on the abdomen.

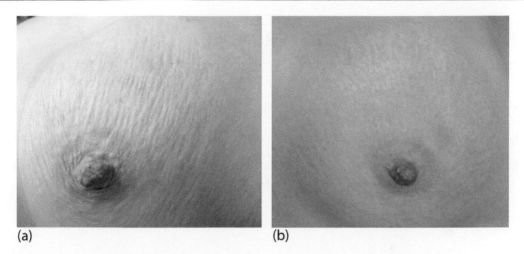

FIGURE 8.11   (a) Breast covered in striae; (b) after one session of AC.

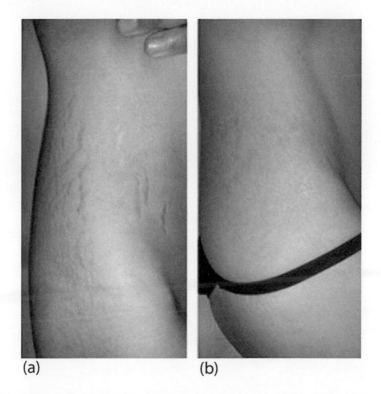

FIGURE 8.12   (a) Striae on the body; (b) after two AC treatments, about 45 days later. (Courtesy of Dr Nenad Stanković, DMD, specialist in Cosmetology, ESTERA.RS.)

REFERENCES

1. Deprez P, Treating the neck and decolletage, in: *Textbook of chemical peels*, second edition, CRC Press, Boca Raton, 2016: 144–151.
2. Deprez P, Treating aging skin of the hands and forearms, in: *Textbook of chemical peels*, second edition, CRC Press, Boca Raton, 2016: 136–143.
3. Deprez P, Face and hands: Actinic keratoses and lentigines, in: *Textbook of chemical peels*, second edition, CRC Press, Boca Raton, 2016: 183–197.
4. Deprez P. Stretch marks, scars and pilar keratosis: Anterior chemabrasion, in: *Textbook of chemical peels*, second edition, CRC Press, Boca Raton, 2016: 152–182.

A Special Note on Some Common Skin Conditions

9

SUN DAMAGE AND LENTIGINES (1,2)

Sun damage has already been discussed in depth, and we have already looked at how we can remove lentigines with focal deep TCA peels. I just wanted to add a word of caution here. Not all lentigines are just benign lentigines! If you ever have ANY doubt about whether a lesion is benign or malignant or require a second opinion from a colleague who is more proficient in dermoscopy, please make further inquiries *before* you attempt any treatment. Lentigo maligna and lentigo malignant melanoma must not be treated with chemical peels without prior consultation with a specialist dermatologist.

Similarly, make sure you do not confuse solar keratoses or seborrhoeic papillomas with BCCs or SCCs.

Please make sure that during the consultation you talk about the importance of sun protection and the meaning of sun avoidance. The presence of a lot of sun damage and lentigines generally means that the patient has had a lot of unprotected sun exposure in the past. Often they will tell you this has not been the case and that they have 'never had sun exposure', but their skin tells a different story. Our role is to educate people so they can look after their skin and prevent sun damage which causes skin ageing and the potential risk of malignancies.

Again, I must emphasize the importance of a good skincare routine. So the preparation phase will allow the patient to get used to this aspect of self-care, and they need to get used to the idea of using sun protection on their face daily, regardless of the weather. I have seen this so often when patients come into the practice, even after a phenol peel, without sun protection, and their excuse is 'I wasn't going out today', or they go and sit in the garden on a sunny day a week or two after a peel and, of course, come in with hyperpigmentation. Sun protection has to be applied every day, even if the patient is not leaving their house. As long as there are windows and daylight comes into their room, there is UV exposure; so it is an absolute must. No matter how much you talk about sun protection and the damage that sun exposure does to the face, it is not enough. So I take every opportunity to do so with my patients.

Nowadays so many great quality total sunscreens are available to us that can easily be used instead of a day moisturizer, and they feel totally non-oily and completely blend in with the skin. Why not get used to the idea of just using it every day on the face?

Figure 9.1 shows some lentigines on the lower cheek on two different patients both with skin type III. Figure 9.2 shows a patient before and after treatment for a lentigo with 15% TCA with a deeper application on the lentigo.

Figure 9.3 shows a patient before and after one medium TCA peel for treatment of sun damage and lentigines.

DOI: 10.1201/9781003244134-9

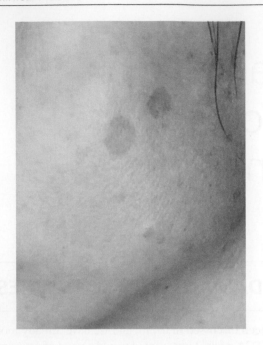

FIGURE 9.1   Lentigines.

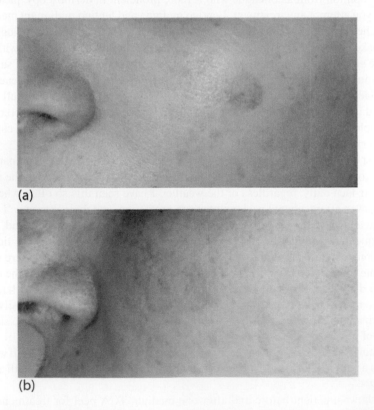

(a)

(b)

FIGURE 9.2   (a) Before and (b) after treatment for a lentigo with 15% TCA with a deeper application on the lentigo. (Courtesy of Dr Nenad Stanković, DMD, specialist in Cosmetology, ESTERA.RS.)

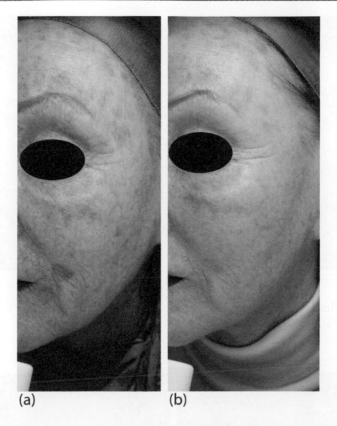

(a)   (b)

FIGURE 9.3   (a) Before and (b) after one medium TCA peel for treatment of sun damage and lentigines.

Figure 9.4 shows a patient before and after 25% TCA treatment, and Figure 9.5 shows a patient before and after 15% TCA treatment.

ACNE

There are plenty of research, protocols, books, articles, and treatment options out there for acne. I just want to give you a simplified and practical version of how to deal with acne in an aesthetic practice, using products and peels (3,4).

Consultation

It is important to gather as much information about the acne history during the consultation. I generally like to go back to earlier years, when acne started. This will give me an idea of whether this is a long-standing issue since the teenage years or more recent. So how long have they suffered from acne?

Then we need to ask about the severity of acne. How bad is it normally? Is today a good day? An average day? Or a bad day? How much does it fluctuate? Does it follow a pattern such as the menstrual cycle in female patients? Are the lesions usually the same type, or have there been any episodes where they have got a lot worse or better?

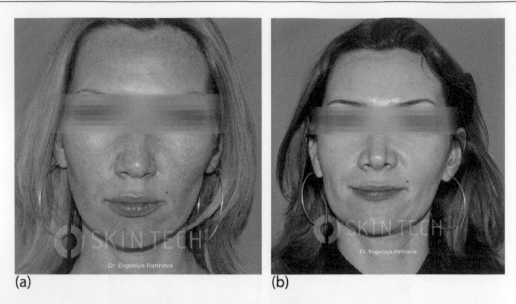

(a)   (b)

FIGURE 9.4   (a) Before and (b) after 25% TCA treatment (using Unideep SkinTech). (Courtesy of Dr Evgeniya Ranneva, PhD, dermatologist, Spain, and Skin Tech Pharma Group.)

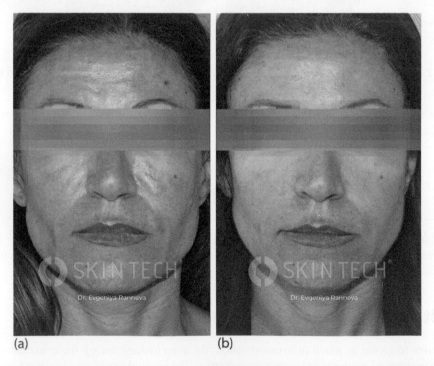

(a)   (b)

FIGURE 9.5   (a) Before and (b) after 15% TCA treatment (using Easy TCA Pain Control SkinTech). (Courtesy of Dr Evgeniya Ranneva, PhD, dermatologist, Spain, and Skin Tech Pharma Group.)

Then the extent of the acne. Does it only affect the face or the body as well? Does it affect the neck, shoulders, or upper back area? If it only affects the face, which part of the face is most affected?

Does their skin generally feel oily, combination, normal, or dry?

Then I want to know every single acne treatment that has ever been used or prescribed by any doctors. So any past courses of oral antibiotics, oral isotretinoin, topicals such as benzoyl peroxide, antibiotics, tretinoin, etc.

You would be surprised how many patients simply do not remember what remedies have been tried so far. Some don't even remember past courses of isotretinoin and it's only on further questioning that they suddenly 'remember'.

Then I want to know exactly which products are used, and in which order, by the patient day and night. Some acne sufferers have no skincare routine whatsoever because they are afraid of putting anything on their skin. Some have very complicated routines and use far too many products, and some over-cleanse their face to reduce the oiliness, which of course ends up being counter-productive.

Also remember to ask about current medication. Are they currently taking a course of antibiotics? Are they on any other non-acne-related medication? Do they take any form of contraception?

Have they ever taken anabolic steroids? Steroid acne is nowadays very common in young gym-goers as anabolic steroids can easily be accessed through individuals in gyms.

What do they do for work? Is their work environment hot? Do they sweat a lot at work? Is the environment dirty? Do they come in contact with any substances that could potentially cause acne? I have seen a few cases of chlorine-induced acne. Very rare but chronic chlorine exposure can cause comedomal acne in adults.

Examination and Assessment

Examine the skin without makeup. Sometimes you need to bring the patient back for this as they are 'unable' to remove their makeup because they have a work meeting after your appointment or are 'going out'. Examining skin covered in makeup – especially foundation – is a waste of time, so I would rather rebook for the patient to come back when they can be without makeup, which allows us to take some digital pictures as well.

Look for the severity of acne. Is it mild, moderate, or severe?

Also look for the lesions present. Are there comedomes? Open comedomes? Closed comedomes? Are there papules? Are there pustules? Usually a combination of these lesions is visible; however, one or two lesion types can sometimes pre-dominate, which determines the type of acne.

Examine the upper body if the acne extends to the non-facial areas.

Look out for any cysts or nodules.

Skincare Recommendations

You cannot treat acne with just medication or just peels or lasers without a skincare routine. It is very important to ensure a good anti-acne skincare routine is in place first. Patients with severe acne are not candidates for peels. Their acne has to be controlled first, which often requires a course of isotretinoin. Anyone who has had a course of isotretinoin should not have any peels or lasers for at least six months after stopping the treatment, as otherwise there is too much risk of damage and scarring.

Please refer to Chapter 5 on skin preparation for some general considerations.

Always remember to write down the skincare routine for the patient step by step and also according to day and night. Use your experience and product knowledge according to the product ranges that you use in your practice. Don't be afraid to use products from different brands in combination; also adapt and adjust the skincare to the patient's skin type and needs.

Start with a good cleanser. This has to be used twice daily. Always use cleansers that need to be washed off with water. Cleansers containing salicylic acid or AHA-BHA combinations are really great for acne-prone skin. This ensures a proper deep cleanse without over-drying the skin and damaging the lipid layer.

If you are going to use a toner after the cleansing step, again choose a toner with BHA or AHA-BHA combinations. Some toners contain AHA-retinoid combinations which are more suitable for nighttime use. Avoid any cleansers that contain alcohol.

The next step is moisturization. Use either use a light serum for this step or a light cream, again preferably containing BHA or BHA-AHA. Avoid any moisturizers with mineral oil; any products used have to be non-comedogenic and oil-free.

Do not forget to recommend a light but high-factor sunscreen. Avoid any heavy oil-based sunscreens.

Always check with your female patients which makeup products they use. Ask them to stop any heavy oil-based makeup and foundation and swap them to pure mineral makeup, which may or may not be liquid. Nowadays there are amazing brands of mineral makeup out there that give plenty of options.

For nighttime I always recommend a retinoid. I think retinoate, retinol, or tretinoin all have a great effect on acne. Warn the patient that their skin may become a bit red and dry and flaky initially, but that will settle down after a few weeks.

Avoid any heavy moisturizers and the typical night creams in acne-prone patients.

Benzoyl peroxide is useful in treating acne. It is best used in the daytime, as it should not be used at the same time as a retinoid. It is an anti-microbial/exfoliating agent. It is best applied to the skin after cleansing and toning and before any creams are applied. The problem with this product is that it stings and burns after application and can cause a lot of irritation and dryness, so a lot of patients find it difficult to stay compliant in the long term.

Hydroquinone (HQ) and/or other tyrosinase inhibitors can be used for acne in darker skin types where a lot of PIH is involved. Please see further the section about PIH. These agents are best used twice daily for best results and, of course, with added sun protection for daytime.

The combination of HQ and retinoids has a remarkable evening-out effect on the skin.

Superficial Peel Recommendations

Numerous peels can be used to treat mild to moderate acne. Simply a course of glycolic acid peels or any AHA combinations will always help. Mandelic acid is often used as an AHA combination with glycolic acid to treat acne because of its anti-acne properties.

Another peel that would work very well is BHA or salicylic acid. This peel would be extremely good for oily skin types and has a good anti-inflammatory effect as well.

Retinol peels are also very useful for treating acne, especially comedomal acne.

Light TCA peels are also very good at clearing acne. However, patients need to be warned about more visible desquamation compared to the previously mentioned peels.

Figure 9.6 shows a patient with papulopustular acne. A full consultation will help to specifically look at every aspect of the problem. It will help to use the Observ filter, as this method of taking photographs will help to assess the extent of the problem, including any PIH and skin congestion.

Figure 9.7 shows another patient with papulopustular acne on the cheek before and after a TCA 15% medium peel. Visibly there is a great level of improvement; however, with the Observ filter (Figure 9.8) the extent of the problem is more noticeable. We can see that there is improvement; however, there is still some work to be done to completely improve the condition. Another medium peel will need to be organized about a month after the first one.

Figure 9.9 shows the result of a course of four superficial TCA 15% peels to treat acne.

Figure 9.10 shows the results for acne treatment with 15% TCA after two treatments a week apart.

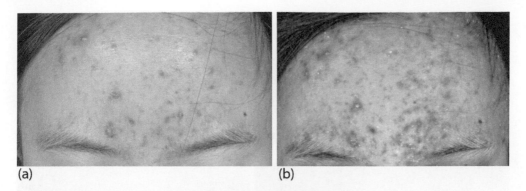

FIGURE 9.6 (a) Papulopustular acne; (b) the same patient viewed with the Observ filter.

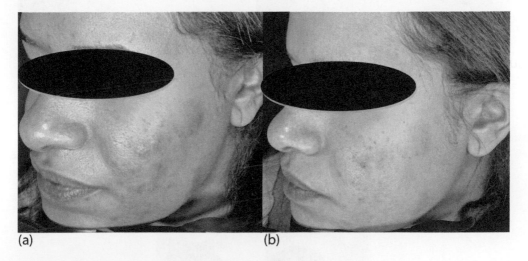

FIGURE 9.7 (a) Before and (b) after a TCA peel for papulopustular acne.

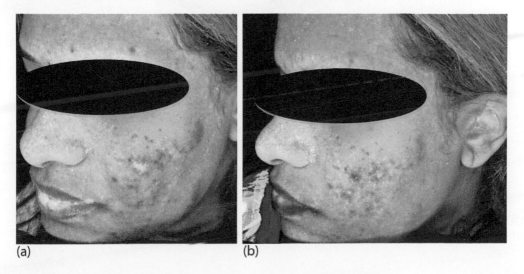

FIGURE 9.8 The same patient as in Figure 9.7, viewed with the Observ filter.

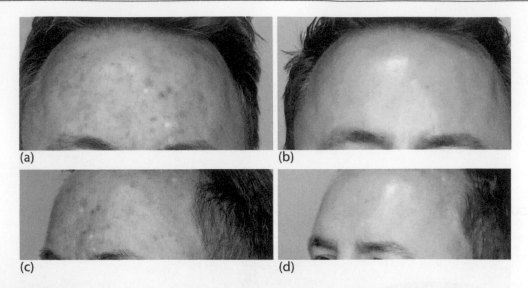

(a)   (b)

(c)   (d)

FIGURE 9.9   (a, c) Before and (b, d) after four superficial TCA 15% peels to treat acne.

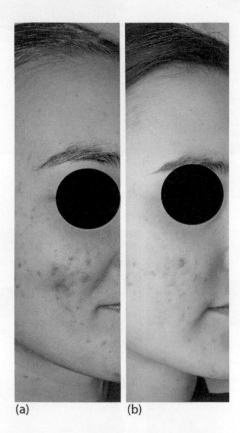

(a)   (b)

FIGURE 9.10   (a) Before and (b) after two treatments with 15% TCA one week apart. (Courtesy of Dr Nenad Stanković, DMD, specialist in Cosmetology, ESTERA.RS.)

Supplements (5)

There are plenty of textbooks about nutritional supplements and how one can improve the skin by taking the correct supplementation or eating the best diet. What we eat certainly does show up on our skin. Having a good diet containing plenty of vitamins and minerals will certainly support our skin. There are two specific supplements I would like to discuss here briefly that can specifically help with acne or in fact any inflammatory skin diseases.

One is probiotics and prebiotics: probiotics are the good bacteria and the prebiotics are the nutritious fibres that help the probiotics grow and proliferate. Having a healthy gut will ensure optimal absorption of nutrients and increase skin health generally. I would recommend a daily intake of pro and prebiotics to improve gut health and nutrient absorption.

The other one is omega-3 fatty acids: each cell in our body, including our skin cells, is made of a cell wall that consists of fatty acids. There are three types of fatty acids, namely omega-3, omega-6, and omega-9. The health of each cell virtually depends on how much omega-3 is present in the cell wall. Omega-3 fatty acids are anti-inflammatory and make the cell wall more flexible. Omega-6 fatty acids are pro-inflammatory and create a rigid cell wall. The balance between these two types of fatty acids will determine how inflamed or how healthy each cell is. The ideal ratio between omega 6-3 is equal or less than 3-1. So for each omega-3 molecule we would ideally have one to three omega-6 molecules. Unfortunately, in over 95% of the global population this is not the case and that is because we do not consume enough foods with active stable omega-3 fatty acids in them. Having a high level of omega-3 will improve any inflammation including acne. The problem is that the majority of available omega-3 supplements on the market are not stable enough to deliver the benefits. Omega-3 supplements have to be accompanied by polyphenols to keep them in their active stable form. Without the polyphenol the fatty acid itself will go rancid and will have very little effect.

Severe Acne Scarring (6,7)

Severe acne scarring is always difficult to treat. First, the acne itself has to be brought under control. The scarring can be improved with peels, but other resurfacing procedures should also be considered.

It is important to assess the type of scarring first.

Ice pick scars can be very small but are very deep and have very sharp edges. This type of scar is impossible to remove with any chemical peel and needs to be excised first.

Box scars are shallow scars that have sharp edges. They can certainly be improved with chemical peels but might not completely disappear. If you gently stretch the scar between two fingers you will see that it becomes more shallow but the edges are still visible. This is how you can recognize a box scar. Sometimes it is also best to perform a subcision to detach the base of the scar from the deeper layers of the dermis before the peel.

Rolling scars are shallow and have no sharp edges. So upon stretching between two fingers they more or less disappear. These are the best type of scars to treat and they will definitely improve with chemical peels.

Pigmented scars: in darker skin types a lot of acne scarring goes hand in hand with the localized PIH occurring around the acne and the scars. This should be treated with appropriate anti-tyrosinase products to achieve the best results.

Naturally, most people might have a combination of these types of scars. So it is best to assess the face in sections to identify where the majority of the scars are and which types are predominant.

Peel Recommendations

To improve severe acne scarring one should look beyond superficial peels. Even though a course of superficial TCA peels will improve it to some degree, generally deeper and more aggressive treatments are required.

Medium TCA peels would certainly improve rolling scars and some box scars and, of course, any pigmentation.

To go deeper one might consider phenol; however, phenol appears to be a lot more powerful when it comes to treating wrinkles and tightening the skin than when treating acne scarring. Obviously, a full-face deep phenol with occlusion would most certainly improve scarring, but there are two other options to consider.

One is a medium TCA pixel peel, which was discussed in earlier chapters. The advantage of this peel is that only the areas of the face that have acne scarring have to be treated with the microneedling first; the rest of the face will just receive a medium TCA. The other advantages are a much shorter treatment time; much less downtime for the patient and no social isolation; much less risk of side effects; it is much better tolerated and less painful compared to a full-face phenol peel; and, of course, it can be repeated. I have to admit this is my favourite peel option for acne scarring (8).

Another option would be an anterior chemoabrasion on the face in the areas with acne scarring (Figures 9.11, 9.12, 9.13). Again this is easier to do than a phenol peel on the whole face and has a much shorter treatment time; however, the areas that have been abraded will need to be covered with BSG powder for a week, so it is not that easy to hide when going out shopping or going to work.

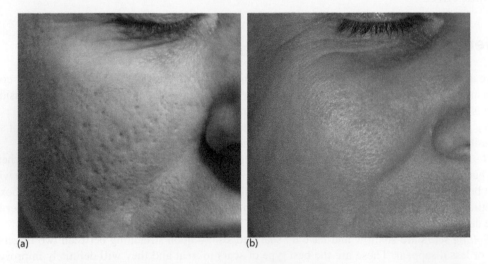

(a)   (b)

FIGURE 9.11   (a) Acne scarring; (b) one year on from three anterior chemabrasion procedures. (Courtesy of Dr Nenad Stanković, DMD, specialist in Cosmetology, ESTERA.RS.)

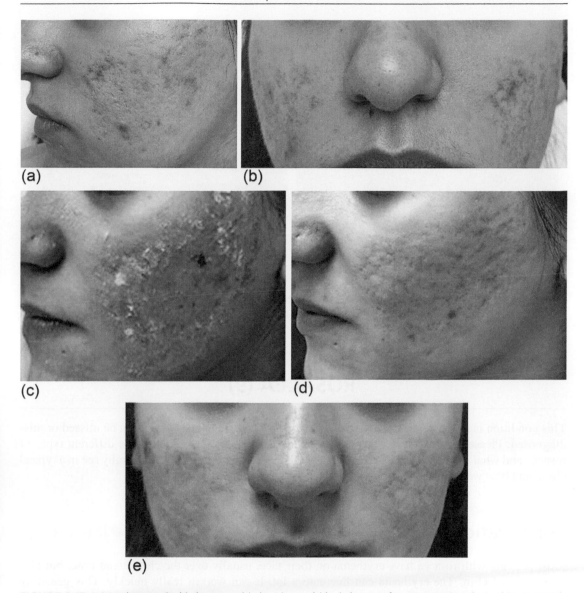

FIGURE 9.12   A patient on (a, b) day zero, (c) day six, and (d, e) day 14 after an anterior chemabrasion with 15% TCA for acne scarring. (Courtesy of Dr Bibiana Romero Otero, Aesthetic Medicine, Brussels.)

The bottom line is we have to always weigh the benefits and the risks of any procedure and also discuss the required downtime with the patient. I would rather have to repeat a less risky procedure and get gradual improvement rather than going too aggressive initially, causing a lot of downtime and still not getting 100% satisfaction. Acne scarring is not easy to treat; I would much rather treat wrinkles.

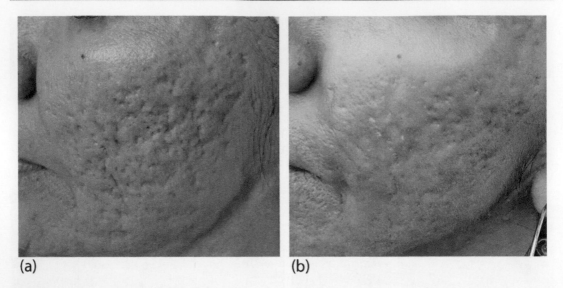

(a)   (b)

FIGURE 9.13   A patient on (a) day zero and (b) day 26 after an anterior chemabrasion with 15% TCA for acne scarring. (Courtesy of Dr Bibiana Romero Otero, Aesthetic Medicine, Brussels.)

ROSACEA (9)

This condition is much more common than we actually think it is. It can also often be missed or misdiagnosed. Please refer to any dermatology textbook to read in detail about all the different types of rosacea and what might be causing it; I am just going to focus here on what we generally see in a typical clinic and how we can help.

Consultation

Most patients with rosacea have erythema on their face, usually over the cheeks and nose, but also forehead and chin. The erythema can fluctuate a lot. It can worsen really quickly. This generally happens if the person gets hot, or emotional, or maybe eats spicy food, or has an alcoholic drink. It can be quite uncomfortable as the person can literally feel their face getting red and hot, and this can sometimes also cause stinging and burning. Often multiple telangiectasias are visible in these areas on the face.

During your consultation, consider the age and gender of the patient. Most people with rosacea are female and middle-aged; however, anyone can suffer from this condition. Ask questions about when the erythema gets worse and what triggers it.

Sometimes rosacea can lead to papules or pustules. There can be multiple lesions present on the face at the same time in different areas. These lesions feel different to typical acne. Your patient can sometimes feel the lesion coming on even before it appears. The papules are very erythematous and feel hard and can cause considerable swelling. They feel painful and sensitive. Not all papules will lead to pustules. Often they just gradually disappear but may take a long time to do so. Therefore this type of rosacea can often be misdiagnosed as acne; however, there are usually no comedomes to see in patients with rosacea.

Examination and Assessment

Things to look out for are general erythema of the face; telangiectasia, especially on the cheeks and nose; and possibly any papules or pustules. Sometimes only one or two lesions are visible, and sometimes there are multiple lesions at the same time. Additionally, the skin itself can often look a bit dry and feel sensitive.

Skincare Recommendations

Rosacea can be improved a lot with good skincare alone. Obviously more serious cases will need oral treatment and even isotretinoin is sometimes given to treat this condition. Low-dose isotretinoin seems to be quite effective as well, but this is outside of the remit of this book.

For cleansers, I would still recommend a wash-off cleanser unless the patient's skin is extremely dry or very sensitive and burns in contact with anything. It is best to remove any makeup or anti-redness concealers with gentle chemical-free makeup wipes first and then cleanse the face. I would prefer to even wash off milk-based cleansers just so that no residue is left on the skin.

I often recommend metronidazole gel or cream as the second step after cleansing. It seems to be quite effective at maintaining the skin in milder cases.

Feel free to use any serums after the metronidazole gel and then follow with a calming and soothing moisturizer.

Do not forget a high-factor SPF cream. Rosacea typically gets worse with sun exposure, so having a good sun protection layer on the face is very important.

At nighttime you could actually use a retinoid if the skin can tolerate it, and of course, you could start at a very low dose and gradually build up. I would still recommend using a soothing moisturizer after the retinoid.

Supplementation

Again I would strongly recommend a highly active poly-phenol-enriched omega-3 supplement. If taken long term, it will improve the condition greatly.

Feel free to also add in the usual prebiotics and probiotics to increase gut health.

Peel Recommendations

There isn't really any specific peel that will 'cure' rosacea. Light peels such as AHA peels will certainly improve the skin's general condition and also help to stimulate and strengthen the skin. TCA superficial or medium peels can be used to help exfoliate the skin much more thoroughly. We just always need to remember that rosacea sufferers generally have more sensitive skin and might not wish to have any aggressive treatments on their face due to the fear of exacerbating the condition. Additionally, due to the dryness of the skin any peel may actually penetrate more deeply than usually expected and cause side effects.

So for the rosacea itself I would recommend gentle peels rather than anything too aggressive.

POST-INFLAMMATORY HYPERPIGMENTATION (10,11)

Post-inflammatory hyperpigmentation (PIH) is a very common problem in skin types IV and above and can sometimes even occur in type III. The skin reacts to inflammation by creating extra pigment in that area. This could be caused by anything that causes injury to the skin, for example, acne spots, a cut or graze, a burn, a chemical peel, a laser, etc.

Consultation

During the consultation ask a lot of questions to see if you can pinpoint a cause; however, most patients will come to see you because they have seen the PIH appear after an event, maybe a treatment or injury, and they know exactly what the cause was.

In darker skin types most acne sufferers will have some degree of PIH accompanying the acne itself. This can make the acne or acne scarring appear a lot worse than it actually is. PIH tends to take a long time to disappear if not treated, so it definitely will mean an accumulation of pigmented spots where the acne has already cleared up.

PIH after treatments is very common; in particular, light-based devices and chemical peels can cause this. The best thing to do is to prepare the skin really well before the procedure and also to make sure that sun protection is in place 100% of the time. PIH can be avoided specifically with chemical peels by carefully selecting the preparation products and also by prolonging the preparation phase as discussed before.

Darker skin types have to be approached with caution even with a longer preparation time. Medium TCA peels are possible on even skin type VI; however, please make sure that you have enough experience with your product and know how to use your peel and what its limitations are.

Examination and Assessment

PIH is typically quite superficial and well demarcated. It often directly mimics the area that was damaged, such as the area of a pustule on the face, or the exact shape of the laser head, or an exact copy of where a peel was applied. Sometimes you can even see which areas were treated first and how deeply each area was treated. I have had a few referrals over the years of terrible cases of PIH on the face after chemical peels.

You could always try and stretch the skin gently between two fingers to see if the pigment lightens a bit. This generally indicates that the pigment is more superficial.

It is important to take good-quality photographs before treating PIH. I would also recommend a Wood's lamp examination or the use of any of the modern cameras that take pictures with different light settings such as the Observ or the Visia system. This is really useful to see the extent of the problem but also to document the progress of the treatment.

Skincare Recommendations

Fortunately, most PIH luckily disappears with a good skincare routine with skin-lightening agents and sun protection (Figure 9.12).

I would include the following in my list of skincare recommendations to suggest as a day and night routine.

For daytime: always anti-oxidants, especially Vitamin C, but also ferulic acid. An AHA combination of – for example – glycolic acid, phytic acid, kojic acid, and lactic acid. Possibly a retinoid-like substance such as bakuchiol. Possibly a tyrosinase inhibitor like hydroquinone. And of course plenty of broad-spectrum sun protection.

For nighttime: always a retinoid such as tretinoin, retinol, or retinoate. Possibly combined with a combination of tyrosinase inhibitors.

Peel Recommendations

Superficial peels would be suitable for this condition if a peel is required. Often the PIH will disappear with the skincare routine; however, if it does persist beyond ten weeks I would suggest a course of superficial peels. These could be AHA- or TCA-based peels.

MELASMA (12–14)

Melasma is a reaction of the skin where the skin creates excessive pigment in very well-demarcated areas of the face. Melasma only affects the face and never body parts, unlike PIH which can appear on any area of the body and face. Generally melasma is caused by a combination of sun exposure and changes in hormones such as pregnancy or use of contraception or the use of UV-sensitizing drugs such as oral retinoids. The patient is most likely to be female, although I have seen one or two cases of men with melasma. This condition is often seen in skin types IV and above, although I have seen it in skin type III as well.

Melasma tends to be a chronic skin condition and has an inflammatory aspect to it and can involve both the epidermis and dermis. The deeper the melasma, the harder it is to improve it. More severe cases of melasma involve damage to the base membrane and possibly solar elastosis.

Consultation

The patients will often have had this problem for a while and most have no idea why they have suddenly developed these pigmented patches on their face. In your consultation it is really important to try and pinpoint when the problem occurred and what may have caused it by asking lots of questions. Sometimes it can be difficult as the problem has been present for years, but in most cases a cause can be identified as explained above.

Unfortunately, melasma is a very difficult and stubborn condition to get rid of and can actually reoccur much later down the line. So I am always very honest with my patients from the onset: I tell them that I believe they have melasma and I explain what the problem is. I also tell them that it is very likely that we will be able to improve the condition and possibly even get rid of it, but there are no guarantees. Even if melasma clears up with skincare products or peels, it can always come back and it often does. It may literally take one holiday or a few days of sun exposure after a successful treatment to bring it out again. So this condition does require a lifetime of maintenance to keep it at bay.

Examination and Assessment

The pigmentation in this case is again very well-demarcated but can be deeper than PIH, so stretching the skin may not lighten the pigment.

The areas most commonly affected are the top lip, the cheeks, and the forehead. Melasma can come in small patches or be very extensive (Figures 9.14, 9.15, 9.16).

Skincare Recommendations

A lot of patients who come in with melasma expect me to give them a magic peel to make it all go away, so they are very surprised when I tell them that their treatment is going to start with a minimum six weeks of skincare. This is the absolute minimum; often these patients will need a routine of at least 12–18 weeks before any procedures can be considered. Often to their surprise the problem dramatically improves with just the products.

For daytime: similar to products recommended for PIH, always anti-oxidants, especially Vitamin C, but also ferulic acid. An AHA combination of, for example, glycolic acid, phytic acid, kojic acid, and lactic acid. Possibly a retinoid-like substance such as bakuchiol. And most definitely a tyrosinase inhibitor like hydroquinone. And, of course, plenty of broad-spectrum sun protection.

For nighttime: always a retinoid such as tretinoin, retinol, or retinoate. Always combined with a tyrosinase inhibitor such as hydroquinone and or others.

The combination of a retinoid with tyrosinase inhibitors such as HQ has a dramatic blending effect on the skin. These ingredients seem to work synergistically to improve pigmentation.

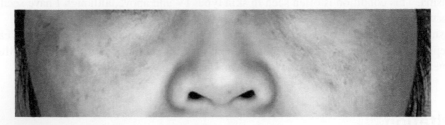

FIGURE 9.14   A typical example of melasma on the cheeks on skin type IV.

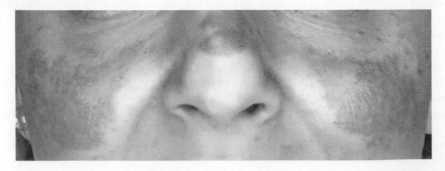

FIGURE 9.15   Another very good example of melasma on the cheeks and on the nose on skin type V.

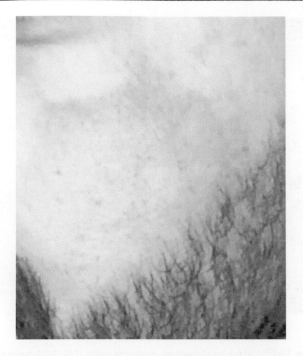

FIGURE 9.16   Melasma on the cheek of a male with skin type V.

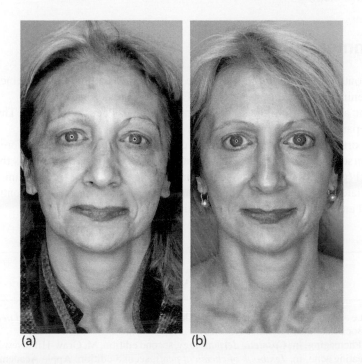

(a)   (b)

FIGURE 9.17   (a) Before and (b) about six months after a 60% phenol peel on the full face to treat skin laxity and melasma. Skin preparation and aftercare with tyrosinase inhibitors are crucial to ensure good results.

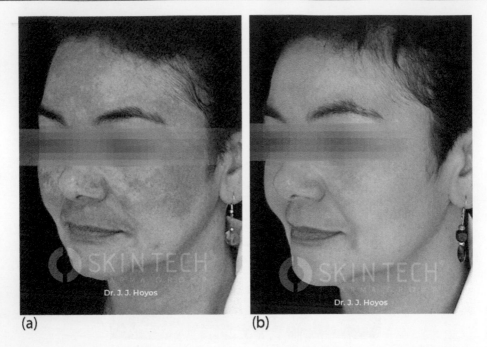

(a)   (b)

FIGURE 9.18   (a) Before and (b) after treatment of melasma with 15% TCA (using Easy TCA SkinTech) and antityrosinase skincare prep (Blending and Bleaching cream SkinTech). (Courtesy of Dr John Jairo Hoyos, aesthetic doctor, Colombia.)

Peel Recommendations

As already mentioned, the condition may improve dramatically with the above skincare routine; however, a peel may enhance the result even further (Figures 9.17 and 9.18).

Make sure the absolute minimum skin preparation time has been adhered to. The darker the skin, the longer the preparation time should be.

It is very important to stop any retinoids or hydroquinone a good five days before the peel. I would recommend a course of superficial TCA peels or a medium TCA peel. As soon as the skin has recovered after the peel (generally day five for superficial TCA and day eight for medium TCA), the patient should go immediately back to using the preparation phase skincare products to continue the improvement and to avoid any worsening of the pigmentation.

REFERENCES

1. Deprez P, Face and hands: Actinic keratoses and lentigines, in: *Textbook of chemical peels*, second edition, CRC Press, Boca Raton, 2016: 183–197.
2. Baumann L, Photoaging, in: *Cosmetic dermatology*, second edition, McGraw-Hill, New York, 2009: 34–41.
3. Deprez P, Treating acne, in: *Textbook of chemical peels*, second edition, Apple Academic Press Inc., Boca Raton, 2016: 126–131.
4. Baumann L, Acne, in: *Cosmetic dermatology*, second edition, McGraw-Hill, New York, 2009: 121–127.

5. Baumann L, Nutrition and the skin, omega-3 fatty acids, in: *Cosmetic dermatology*, second edition, McGraw-Hill, New York, 2009: 56–57.
6. Deprez P, Stretch marks, scars and pilar keratosis: Anterior chemabrasion, in: *Textbook of chemical peels*, second edition, CRC Press, Boca Raton, 2016: 152–182.
7. Baumann L, Facial scar revision, in: *Cosmetic dermatology*, second edition, McGraw-Hill, New York, 2009: 227–223.
8. Deprez P, Combination peels, microneedling pixel peel, in: *Textbook of chemical peels*, second edition, CRC Press, Boca Raton, 2016: 380–382.
9. Baumann L, Rosacea, in: *Cosmetic dermatology*, second edition, CRC Press, Boca Raton, 2016: 128–132.
10. Deprez P, Treatment for hyperpigmentation, in: *Textbook of chemical peels*, second edition, CRC Press, Boca Raton, 2016: 18.
11. Deprez P, Treating melasma, chloasma and postinflammatory hyperpigmentation, in: *Textbook of chemical peels*, second edition, CRC Press, Boca Raton, 2016: 116–125.
12. Deprez P, Treatment for hyperpigmentation, in: *Textbook of chemical peels*, second edition, CRC Press, Boca Raton, 2016: 18.
13. Deprez P, Treating melasma, chloasma and postinflammatory hyperpigmentation, in: *Textbook of chemical peels*, second edition, CRC Press, Boca Raton, 2016: 116–125.
14. Baumann L, Skin pigmentation and pigmentation disorders, in: *Cosmetic dermatology*, second edition, McGraw-Hill, New York, 2009: 98–108.

Mosaic Peels

10

A mosaic peel is when the face is divided into the usual cosmetic subunits, but different peels are applied to different areas. The usual combinations here are TCA and phenol: for example, a light TCA peel with a medium TCA in a specific zone; a medium TCA peel with a light phenol peel in a specific zone; or a medium TCA peel with a deep phenol peel in a specific zone; and finally a light phenol peel with a deep phenol peel in a specific zone.

These combinations will allow you to adjust the peel depth according to the issues or area of concern, without having to go deep all over the face; for example, a patient with moderate sun damage and vertical top lip lines could benefit from a medium TCA full face with a deep phenol peel on the top lip area. Someone who is concerned about peri-orbital skin laxity and wrinkles could have a medium TCA peel full face with a deep phenol peel for both upper and lower eyelids.

Virtually any combination is possible. The SkinTech Lip&Eyelid Formula peel has been specifically designed to be adaptable to these combinations. It can be used in just one area, such as the upper eyelids, or the entire peri-orbital and peri-oral area in combination with a medium TCA peel to even out the peel and blend everything in. Using this technique also allows you to build your confidence by performing a deep peel on small, more manageable areas and gradually progressing to the full face.

I am now going to describe how to do a mosaic peel with a medium TCA full face with the Lip&Eyelid Formula for both the peri-orbital and peri-oral areas. I will describe each step: TCA, upper eye, lower eye, top lip, and bottom lip and chin. You can choose to only treat the upper eyelids, or only the lower eyelids, or just the top lip, or just the lower lip and chin, or any combination that you would like. As long as you use a medium TCA peel over the remaining areas not treated with phenol, you will be able to even the peel out (1).

MEDIUM TCA PEEL

1) Give your patient some oral analgesia 30–45 mins before the peel (for example, an NSAID and/or codeine phosphate).
2) Remove all makeup and cleanse the skin.
3) Cleanse the skin again with your specific pre-peel cleanser.
4) Dry the skin off.
5) Use pure alcohol to fully disinfect the skin all over with a gauze swab.
6) Then use pure acetone to fully degrease the face with a gauze swab.
7) Use a white skin marker to divide the face into 13 different zones (see Figure 7.21).

DOI: 10.1201/9781003244134-10

8) Take out the required amount of your TCA peel into a small dish or bowl. Some formulations require mixing, while others don't. If mixing TCA with a base solution is required, make absolutely sure that you follow the exact instructions of the brand you use to get the correct percentage of the TCA after mixing.

9) Use one or two cotton buds to apply the TCA solution to the face. Make absolutely sure that the cotton buds are not too wet so that the TCA does not drip and run down the face or even worse in the eyes. *This is extremely dangerous.*

   Apply the TCA to the following cosmetic subunits according to Figure 7.21. Once one area is fully covered, then move on to the next area and move around the face to complete the application in all areas.

10) Use a fan to dry the TCA on the skin and cool the face off. TCA application causes stinging and heat and can be quite uncomfortable even at low percentages.

11) There is no need to use a timer as most TCA peels are self-neutralizing and there is no need to remove them. There are, however, exceptions to this rule, so please make sure you follow the instructions according to your specific peel.

12) The expected reaction on the face is full white frosting with a pink background all over the face.

13) If frosting does not appear or a deeper frosting is desired, apply a second coat to all the areas of the face as before and dry and cool off the face with a fan.

14) A full white frost with a pink background indicates that the TCA has penetrated the papillary dermis. The pink background indicates that the dermal blood vessels have not yet been denatured by TCA. At this stage we also notice a papery plastic-like appearance to the skin, which is called epidermal sliding. This is due to the separation of the dermo-epidermal junction.

15) Apply the recommended post-peel recovery cream only to the areas treated with the TCA, making sure none gets onto the untreated areas.

LOWER EYELID PHENOL PEEL

1) When it comes to peeling the eyelids with phenol, I actually prefer to start with the lower eyelids. The logic behind that is that when performing the peel on the lower eyelid, the patient has to keep their eyes open and look up, and I find it is easier to do that first and then ask them to close their eyes and follow with the upper eyelid peel since for that step the eyelids can remain closed.

2) There is no anaesthesia required for peeling the eyelids, as the pain will only last about ten seconds after the peel application. Apply a small amount of ophthalmic Vaseline to the eye, and ask the patient to open and close their eyes a few times to spread the ointment over the eye.

3) Take out the required amount of the product out of the vial into a syringe, and apply the required amount as per your specific peel instructions to your cotton bud. Make absolutely sure it is not dripping wet. *Dripping phenol into the eye is extremely dangerous* and can lead to permanent damage to the eye.

4) Explain to the patient what you are going to do, as you will need their cooperation and you will also need them to stay very calm. Explain to them that you are going to ask them to open their eyes and look up towards their forehead and keep that position until you ask them to

close their eyes. Tell them once you apply the solution under the eyes, it will burn but it will only last for ten seconds.

5) Ask the patient to open their eyes and look up. Use a single cotton bud to apply an even layer of the peel to the entire lower eyelid area. You can go as close as 2mm from the lash line. As soon as you start applying the product, start counting down 10, 9, 8, 7, and so on. This will allow the patient to focus on the counting and makes them less likely to panic and want to close their eyes.

6) By the time you count down to one, a uniform pure white frost has appeared and there is absolutely no burning or pain.

7) Repeat the same process on the other lower eyelid.

8) Allow the initial frosting to disappear. You can now go back to the first eyelid and apply a second layer of the peel following the exact same process. This time the application will be totally pain-free.

9) Repeat the second layer on the other eye.

10) Apply some extra ophthalmic Vaseline to the eyes and ask the patient to close their eyes, ready for the upper eyelid application.

11) Apply the post-peel cream to the lower eyelids, then apply the BSG powder onto the area.

UPPER EYELID PHENOL PEEL

1) This is much easier to do than the lower eyelids because the patient has their eyes shut the whole time.

2) There is no anaesthesia required for peeling the eyelids, as the pain will only last about ten seconds after the peel application. Apply a small amount of ophthalmic Vaseline to the eye and ask the patient to open and close their eyes a few times to spread the ointment over the eye.

3) Take out the required amount of the product out of the vial into a syringe, and apply the required amount as per your specific peel instructions to your cotton bud. Make absolutely sure it is not dripping wet. *Dripping phenol into the eye is extremely dangerous* and can lead to permanent damage to the eye.

4) Ask the patient to keep their eyes shut. Use a single cotton bud to apply an even layer of the peel to the entire upper eyelid area. You can go as close as the tarsus. As soon as you start applying the product, start counting down 10, 9, 8, 7, and so on. This will allow the patient to focus on the counting and makes them less likely to panic.

5) By the time you count down to one, a uniform pure white frost has appeared and there is absolutely no burning or pain.

6) Repeat the same process on the other upper eyelid.

7) Allow the initial frosting to disappear. You can now go back to the first eyelid and apply a second layer of the peel following the exact same process. This time the application will be totally pain-free.

8) Repeat the second layer on the other eye.

9) Apply the post-peel cream to the lower eyelids, then apply the BSG powder onto the area.

10) Make sure there is no BSG powder applied to the tarsus as that will make it difficult for the patient to open their eyes once the BSG sets as crust.

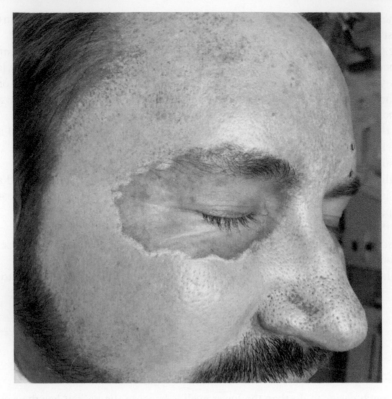

FIGURE 10.1   First stage of a mosaic peel for the eyelids.

Figure 10.1 shows the first stage of a mosaic peel for the eyelids. At this stage the full face has been treated with three coats of 15% TCA, providing a papillary dermis medium-depth TCA peel on the whole face. The 'pink frost' is pretty much uniform.

At the second stage of the peel, namely the application of the phenol peel for the lower eyelids (Figure 10.2), you can clearly see that the pink frost of the medium peel has more or less disappeared, and you can see the pure white frost caused by the 60% phenol peel on the lower eyelid. The next step will be to finish the peel on the upper eyelids and apply the BSG powder around the eyes.

On the day after the peel, the face looks dry and darker than normal due to the medium TCA peel. It has had an application of an aftercare cream (Figure 10.3). The peri-orbital areas are, of course, still covered in the BSG powder and will remain so for seven days.

Figure 10.4 shows a patient being prepared to receive an upper eyelid 60% phenol peel. The face is being cleaned and disinfected first. Lines are then drawn to indicate the area to which to apply the peel (Figure 10.5). Acid is applied to the upper eyelid with one single cotton bud (Figure 10.6), and a white frost appears on the upper eyelid after two coats of the acid (Figure 10.7). Post-peel cream is applied to the area after the peel has been completed (Figure 10.8), and the eyelid is covered with the BSG powder, which will have to stay in place for seven days (Figure 10.9).

The procedure is then repeated for the other eyelid (Figure 10.10), and that eyelid also is now covered in the BSG powder (Figure 10.11).

Figure 10.12 shows the patient on day three after the peel. On day nine (Figure 10.13) healing is complete and the bright red erythema is very visible (as expected) and will take up to 12 weeks to settle down.

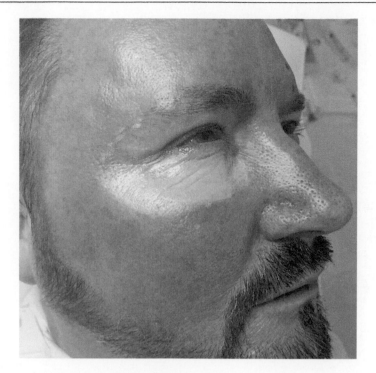

FIGURE 10.2   Second stage of a mosaic peel for the eyelids.

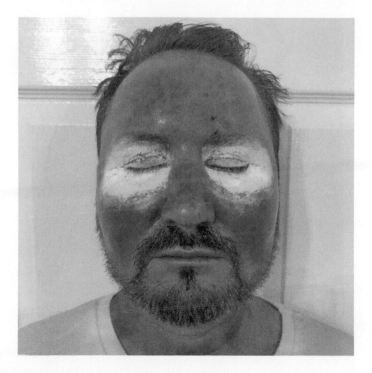

FIGURE 10.3   The day after the mosaic peel for the eyelids.

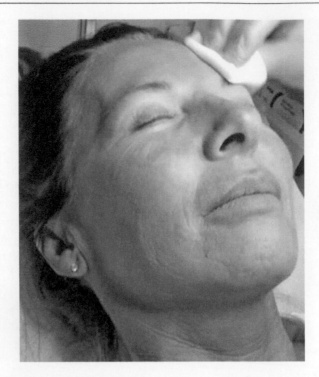

FIGURE 10.4   Patient being cleansed and disinfected before an upper eyelid phenol peel.

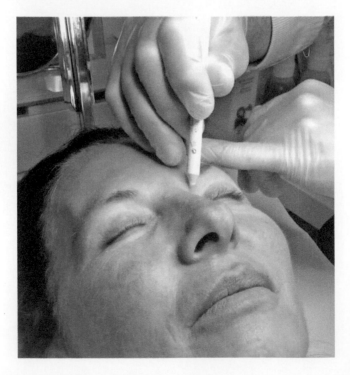

FIGURE 10.5   Marking the area for application.

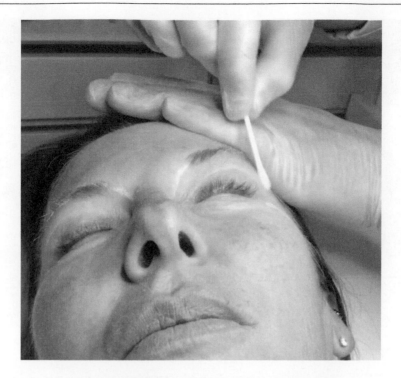

FIGURE 10.6   Application to the upper eyelid.

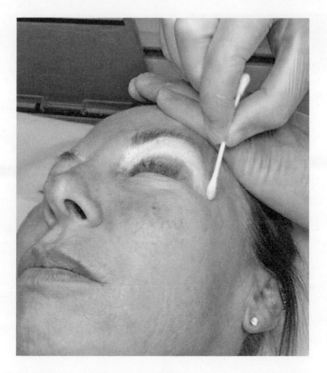

FIGURE 10.7   White first appearing on the upper eyelid.

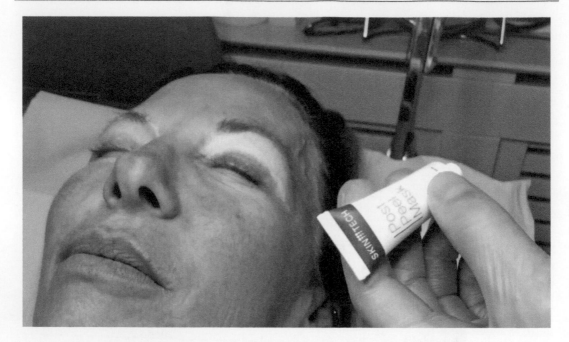

FIGURE 10.8   Application of post-peel cream.

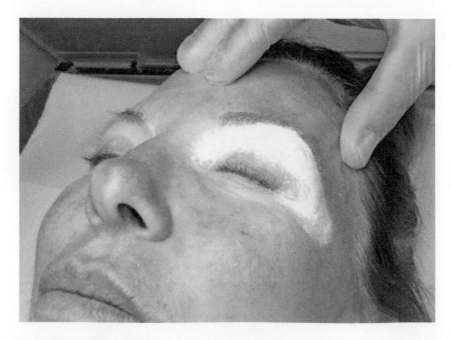

FIGURE 10.9   Eyelid covered with BSG powder.

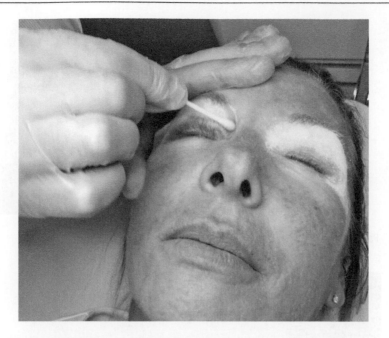

FIGURE 10.10 Starting the procedure on the other eyelid.

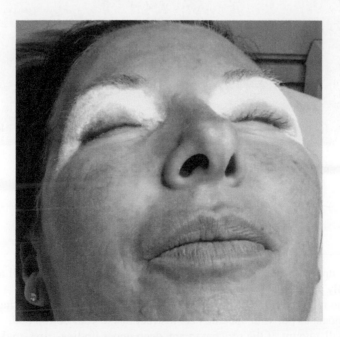

FIGURE 10.11 Both eyelids covered with BSG powder.

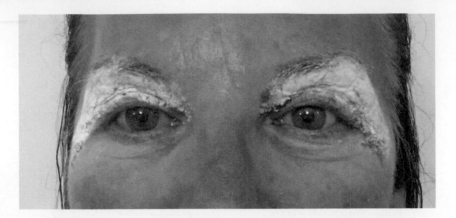

FIGURE 10.12   Patient on day three after the peel.

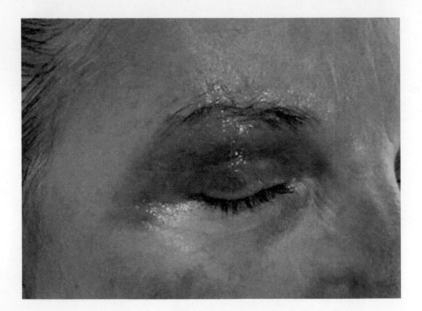

FIGURE 10.13   Patient on day 13 after the peel.

UPPER LIP PHENOL PEEL

1) Perform an upper lip dental infiltration with local anaesthesia. This will allow you to perform a totally painless phenol peel on the upper lip.
2) Take out the required amount of the product out of the vial into a syringe and apply the required amount as per your specific peel instructions to your cotton bud.
3) Apply a small amount of the product to any deep upper lip lines first, making sure that the base of the wrinkles completely frosts.
4) Then start with the application of the first layer to the entire area. A pure white frost should appear over the full area.
5) Allow the frost to disappear and then repeat the process, applying another coat to the entire area.

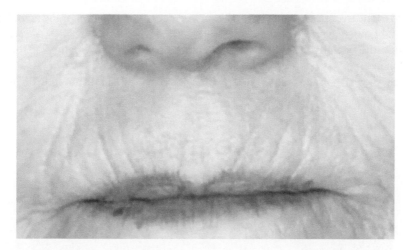

FIGURE 10.14   Patient with peri-oral lines.

6) At this point you have the option to occlude the area or not; occlusion will allow a deeper action of the peel by macerating the epidermis.
7) If not opting for occlusion, just apply the post-peel cream and then apply the BSG powder to the top lip.
8) If occluding, then take your time to apply the occlusive tape to the entire top lip area and ask the patient to avoid facial movements to avoid the tape coming off.
9) The patient will have to return to the clinic the following day so you can remove the occlusive tape and then apply the cream and the BSG powder.

Figure 10.14 shows a patient unhappy with her peri-oral lines who wants resurfacing on the top lip only. For this, 60% phenol was applied on the upper lip alone; two coats of the peel were applied, paying special attention to the upper lip lines. A good solid white-grey frost is visible (Figure 10.15). Occlusive

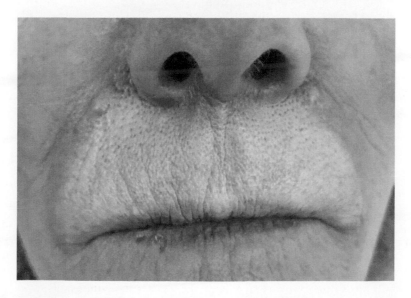

FIGURE 10.15   Two coats of phenol peel applied to the upper lip alone.

tape was applied to the treated area to ensure a better and deeper penetration of the acid. It needs to stay in place for 12–24 hours (Figure 10.16).

The next day the occlusive tape was removed and replaced by application of the BSG powder, which will now stay in place for seven days (Figure 10.17).

Figure 10.18 shows the same patient two weeks later, with a small amount of makeup used to reduce the appearance of the erythema.

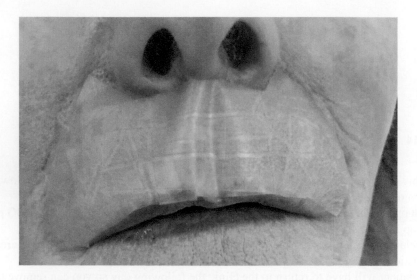

FIGURE 10.16   Occlusive tape is applied.

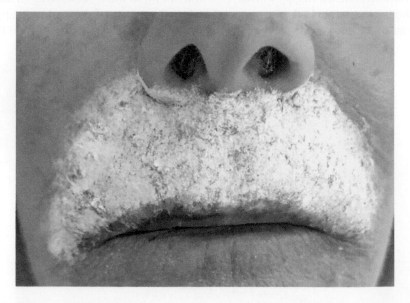

FIGURE 10.17   BSG powder is applied.

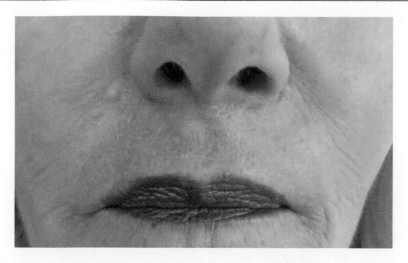

FIGURE 10.18   Result two weeks later.

LOWER LIP AND CHIN PHENOL PEEL

1) Perform a lower lip dental infiltration with local anaesthesia. This will allow you to perform a totally painless phenol peel on the lower lip and is relatively pain-free over the chin area.
2) Take the required amount of the product out of the vial into a syringe, and apply the required amount as per your specific peel instructions to your cotton bud.
3) Apply a small amount of the product to any deep lower lip lines first, making sure that the base of the wrinkles completely frosts.
4) Then start with the application of the first layer to the entire area. A pure white frost should appear over the full area.
5) Allow the frost to disappear and then repeat the process, applying another coat to the entire area.
6) In the chin area one may need to apply a third coat, depending on skin thickness.
7) At this point you have the option to occlude the area or not; occlusion will allow a deeper action of the peel by macerating the epidermis.
8) If not opting for occlusion, just apply the post-peel cream and then apply the BSG powder to the entire area.
9) If occluding, then take your time to apply the occlusive tape to the entire lower lip and chin area, and ask the patient to avoid facial movements to avoid the tape coming off.
10) The patient will have to return to the clinic the following day so you can remove the occlusive tape and then apply the cream and the BSG powder.

Figure 10.19 shows a patient being prepared for a mosaic peel with two types of phenol: 60% phenol for the eyelids and the top lip and 30% phenol for the lower lip/chin and the rest of the face. The first step is cleansing the skin, followed by disinfecting and degreasing with first alcohol, then acetone (Figure 10.20). The face is divided into subunits; in Figure 10.21 I have added a small extra section in the glabella here as the lines were quite deep in this area.

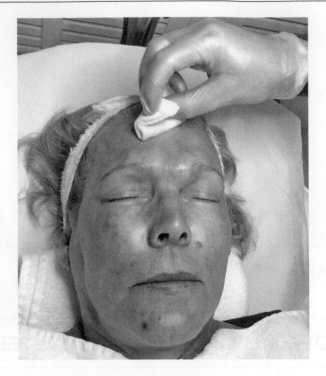

FIGURE 10.19   Cleansing the skin.

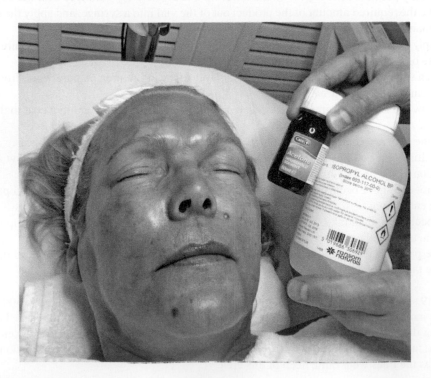

FIGURE 10.20   Disinfecting and degreasing the skin.

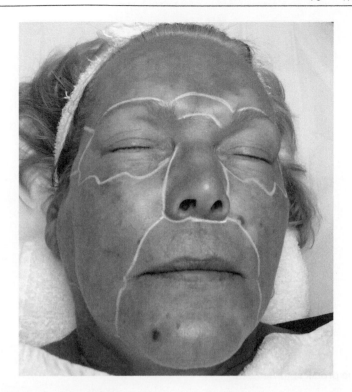

FIGURE 10.21   Marking the facial subunits.

Figure 10.22 shows the two products being used, namely Lip&Eyelid formula (60%) and Easy Phen Light (30%). Acid was applied to the top lip. In Figure 10.23 the white frost is forming; one more coat will be needed to complete this area. Figure 10.24 shows the application of the peel on the lower lip/chin section. Again, a white frost is forming; two to three coats will be needed to get a good level of treatment in this area. Figure 10.25 shows applying the peel on the lower eyelids: the frost is forming and the patient needs to keep looking up so that the entire area right up to the edge of the eyelid can be treated. The peel is then applied to the lower eyelid on the other side; in Figure 10.26 the frosting is now more obvious on both sides. The peel is then applied to the upper eyelids (Figure 10.27). After this step the forehead and the cheeks will be treated one by one with the necessary time gap between each area. Figure 10.28 shows the application of the BSG powder to the full face after the peel has been completed. Figure 10.29 shows the patient immediately after the completion of the procedure.

Figure 10.30 shows the patient on day one after the peel; more BSG powder has been applied to the face. There is not much oedema visible in this case. The patient returned for her day three post-peel review. There are no signs of any complications (Figure 10.31). By the day six review (Figure 10.32) the patient will be able to cover her face with an ointment the following evening, and all the BSG and skin will come off on the morning of day eight.

Figure 10.33 illustrates a mosaic peel of the upper eyelid only: 60% phenol was used on the upper eyelids and three coats of 15% TCA were used for the medium peel on the rest of the face. The picture after the procedure shows the remarkable chemical upper blepharoplasty that has been achieved with this treatment.

Figure 10.34 illustrates a mosaic peel involving a medium TCA peel on the face and 60% phenol on both the upper and lower eyelids. On day one after the mosaic peel the BSG powder protects the

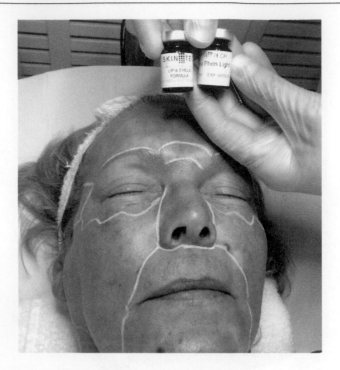

FIGURE 10.22   The products to be used.

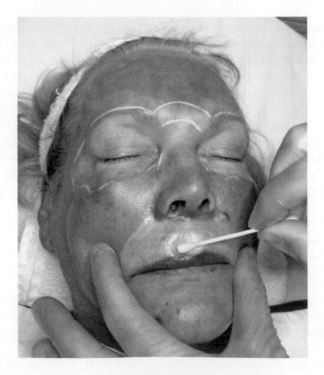

FIGURE 10.23   After one application to the top lip, a white frost is forming.

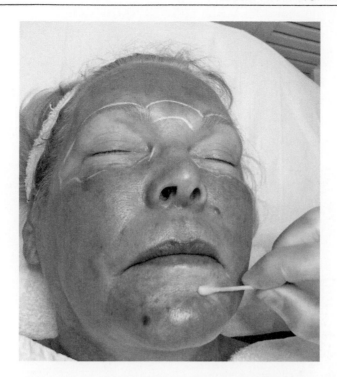

FIGURE 10.24   First application of peel on the lower lip and chin section.

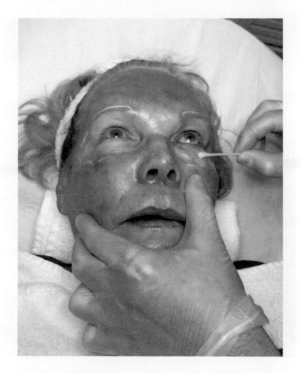

FIGURE 10.25   Applying the peel on the lower eyelid.

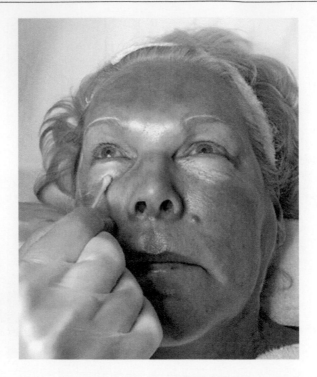

FIGURE 10.26   Applying the peel to the other lower eyelid; frosting is now more obvious on both sides.

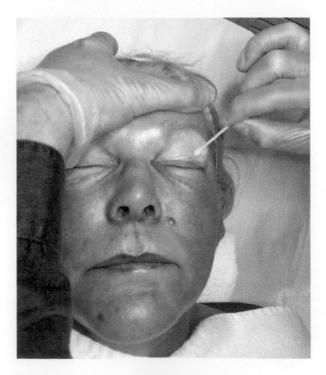

FIGURE 10.27   Applying the peel to the upper eyelids.

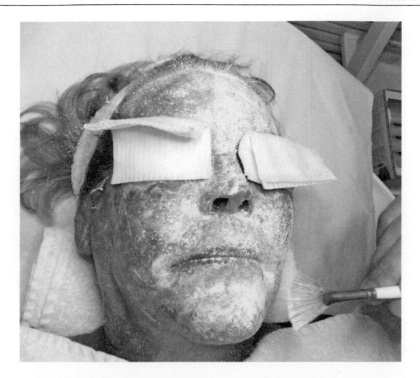

FIGURE 10.28 Applying BSG powder after the peel.

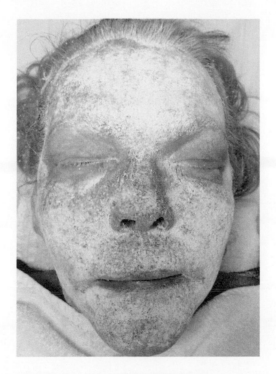

FIGURE 10.29 Patient immediately after completion of the peel.

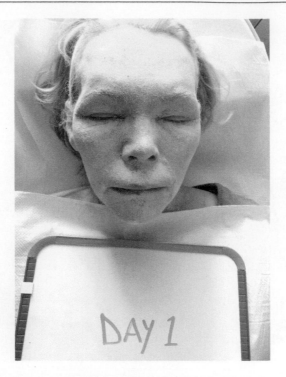

FIGURE 10.30   Patient on day one after the peel.

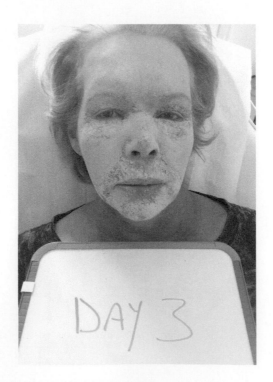

FIGURE 10.31   Patient on day three after the peel.

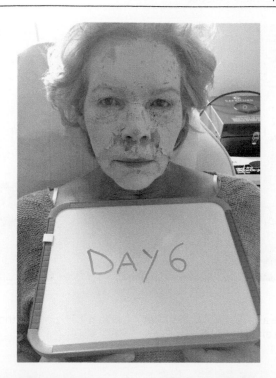

FIGURE 10.32   Patient on day six after the peel.

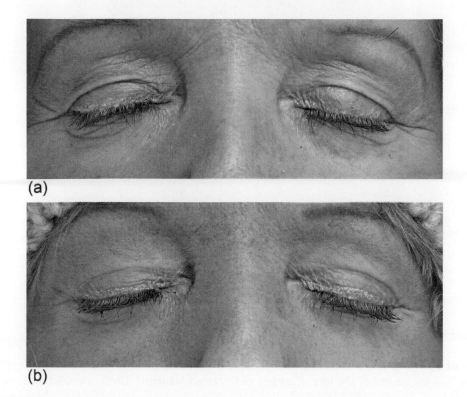

FIGURE 10.33   (a) Before and (b) after a mosaic peel of the upper eyelid only.

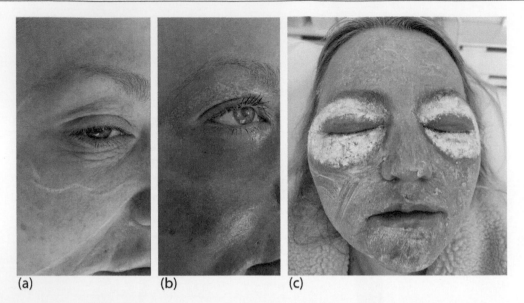

(a)   (b)   (c)

FIGURE 10.34   (a) Before and (b) two weeks after a medium TCA peel on the face and 60% phenol on the eyelids. (c) On day one after the peel.

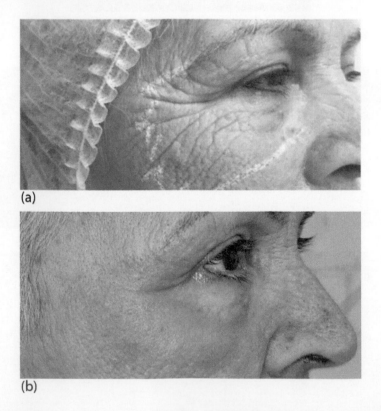

(a)

(b)

FIGURE 10.35   (a) Before and (b) four months after a peel with 60% phenol for the peri-orbital area and 15% TCA on the rest of the face. (Courtesy of Dr Nenad Stanković, DMD, specialist in Cosmetology, ESTERA.RS.)

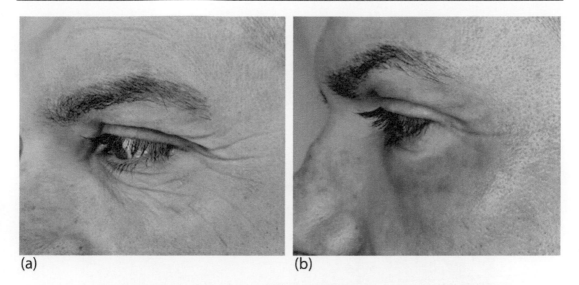

(a)   (b)

FIGURE 10.36   (a) Before and (b) day ten post-peel images for 60% phenol for the peri-orbital area and 15% TCA on the rest of the face. (Courtesy of Dr Nenad Stanković, DMD, specialist in Cosmetology, ESTERA.RS.)

peri-orbital areas while sunscreen has been applied to the rest of the face. The level of oedema is completely normal and will take at least three days to dissipate. After two weeks peri-orbital erythema is still clearly visible and will take at least another four to six weeks to blend in.

Figures 10.35 to 10.37 illustrate mosaic peels with phenol and TCA; Figure 10.38 illustrates the results of a mosaic peel using different types of TCA.

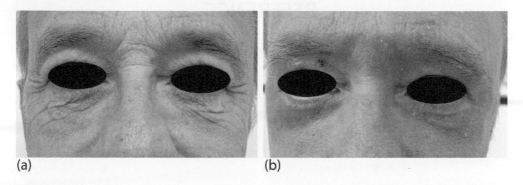

(a)   (b)

FIGURE 10.37   (a) On day zero and (b) day 12 after a mosaic peel with 60% phenol peel in the peri-orbital region and medium TCA peel on the rest of the face. (Courtesy of Dr Bibiana Romero Otero, Aesthetic Medicine, Brussels.)

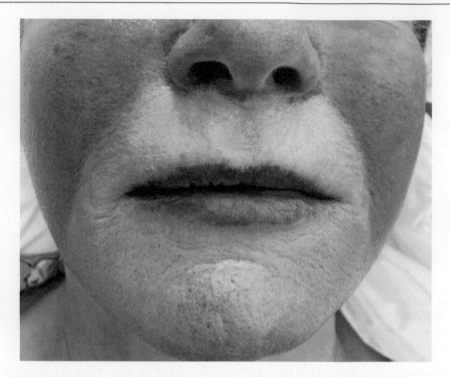

FIGURE 10.38 A mosaic peel using two different types of TCA. The face has been treated with two coats of 15% TCA, while the peri-oral area has been treated with two coats of 25% TCA. The difference in the level of frosting is very obvious. The peri-oral area shows a deep and complete pink frost.

REFERENCE

1. Deprez P, Phenol: Chemical blepharoplasty and cheiloplasty, in: *Textbook of chemical peels*, second edition, CRC Press, Boca Raton, 2016: 307–324.

Aftercare

11

Aftercare is everything! Good and appropriate aftercare after a peel will ensure great skin healing and recovery and reduce the risk of any side effects.

Most mistakes tend to happen at this stage and some patients tend to come up with their own ingenious aftercare protocols, so it is imperative that at this stage they follow what we instruct them to do. With the best will in the world and even when we write down exact aftercare protocols, some will always deviate from them. I prefer to give written aftercare instructions and reiterate the importance of following them to the letter. Two extreme examples of when my patients have deviated from my instructions are: one patient pulled all her skin off her face three days after a medium TCA peel and luckily did not get any side effects. Another patient's mother put Vaseline all over the patient's face on the second day after a phenol peel, when she was told specifically not to use anything else but the BSG powder. Both these patients recovered well without any side effects, but they were lucky; some will not be this lucky and will get problems.

AHA-BHA PEEL AFTERCARE

Usually aftercare after a light epidermal peel is fairly simple. You already know that there is little downtime after such a peel. Downtime can vary from just dry skin to some minor skin desquamation over a period of three to five days. Usually these are not very visible complications and definitely not bad enough to stop anyone from doing anything they would usually do in their life.

However, it is important to bear a few things in mind. It is important to use your after-peel recovery product (whatever that may be, depending on the brand you use) for at least three to five days with additional appropriate high-factor sun protection.

Going back to using the prep phase products immediately after the peel might be too irritating for the skin, so it is always a good idea to let the skin recover for at least a few days, even if there is no visible desquamation at all.

For those skin types at risk of PIH, I would incorporate an anti-tyrosinase product in the after-peel routine and emphasize the importance of sunscreen use and sun avoidance. Remember that even the best high-factor sunscreens will still let UV light through, and a long walk outside or sitting in the garden (even in the shade) immediately after any peel is never a good idea.

After five days the patient can go back to using the prep phase products.

The same principle goes for retinol-based peels; even though there may be slightly more desquamation with these peels, they are still epidermal peels with little downtime.

DOI: 10.1201/9781003244134-11

SUPERFICIAL TCA AFTERCARE

TCA will always have more downtime than a non-TCA-based peel. A basal layer peel on most people might give the same downtime as an AHA or retinol peel but may on others cause more visible desquamation; a Grenz-zone peel will be slightly more visible again. However, this really depends on the skin type and on the level and products used for skin prep in the period running up to the peel.

I would generally instruct the patients to use the post-peel recovery product and their sunscreen for five to seven days after a superficial TCA peel. There should be no other disruption to normal daily activities except a few days of flaky skin.

MEDIUM TCA AFTERCARE

A medium peel is a true peel and needs to be respected as such. With a medium TCA peel the entire skin becomes like a layer of plastic stuck on the surface of the face and will get tighter as the days go by. Here are my tips for aftercare; as someone who has a medium TCA peel every year without fail to maintain the health of my skin, I can speak from experience.

Plan your peel carefully. Look at your diary and consider anything that you have planned for the week following the peel. You will essentially need to have as little as possible to do. Following a medium TCA peel you will not want to socialize or go out too much because you will look and feel uncomfortable. Ideally, you would want to stay home for at least five to six days. If that is not possible, remember that in the first three days after the peel you will not have started peeling yet. Your skin will look like a tight mask, but you can still go out for a bit of essential food shopping or a quick child pick-up from school, but from day four onwards you will be peeling and probably would not want to let anyone see what you look like.

It always makes me smile when people ask me if they can wear makeup after a medium peel. My answer is you can try but it won't make any difference. You need to understand that this is actually a serious procedure and has to be respected as such.

Ask your patient to wash their hair the day before or the morning of the peel (day zero). From day one to day three hair washing is not a good idea. The skin has to stay relatively dry and standing under a hot shower is a very bad idea. On day four after the peel the hair can be washed carefully, allowing the shampoo and water to run back from the forehead towards the neck and shoulders, so still not soaking under a hot shower. Only from day six or seven would I recommend a normal shower with a normal hair wash.

From day one to day six I would recommend a shower from the neck down and never directly over the head or face, unless the hair is being washed as explained above. I would recommend against sitting in a hot bath as that will induce sweating and may lead to sweat blisters forming under the dead layer of skin on the face (which happened to one of my patients).

I would strongly advise patients not to exercise for six days. Sweating has to be kept to an absolute minimum, and the first six days after a medium peel are not the best time for the gym or an outdoor run.

Ask your patient to wash their face gently with a very gentle cleanser (which you, of course, provided in your skincare kit for them) and lukewarm water morning and night. Ask them to apply their post-peel recovery cream immediately after washing and in the morning to follow that with a liberal amount of sunscreen.

Male patients should shave the day before their peel and not shave until day six or seven after the peel. Excessive facial movements should be restricted to a minimum during the first week. Having botulinum toxin a week or two before the peel is actually a very good idea; chewing food, laughing, smiling, yawning – all these movements should be limited to an absolute minimum. Trying to make your skin crack by moving your face or trying to pull faces is a bad idea, as it can cause bleeding and possibly infection or even scarring. Your patient has to understand that under this thin layer of plastic-like dead skin, there is essentially open papillary dermis with zero protection, so it is a very bad idea to remove the dead skin prematurely. They must also resist the temptation of pulling their skin off, even on day five when everything feels like it's about to come off.

Let the skin come off naturally. Most people will have completely peeled by day seven; however, some individuals may still have areas that have yet to peel on days 8–11. The better the skin preparation was prior to the peel, the shorter the peeling phase will be and thus the quicker the recovery time.

PHENOL PEEL AFTERCARE (1)

After a phenol peel the patient always seems to be OK while they are at the clinic. Once they get back home or to their hotel to recover, they often feel an intense burning and pulsating inflammatory pain on the entire face. The analgesia given to them before and after the treatment in combination with the anxiolytics should allow them to calm down and fall asleep and rest. However, this is difficult when dealing with a patient who is panicking and not listening to instructions. My advice is to keep the room really cool and to have a fan at full blast on the face for the next five to seven hours. This really helps the pain as well. After a period of roughly five to eight hours, this pain will stop and there will be no further pain during the recovery time.

The eyes can tear intensely as well and this is normal. As time goes on, the face will swell up and the eyelids will often close completely. If an occlusive mask was applied, then some fluid may form underneath it and drip down the neck, which is completely normal. If no occlusive mask was applied and only BSG powder, then the swelling will be more intense over the entire face.

It is important for the patient to drink plenty through a straw and not forget to take their medication. They will need the help of their supporting person to ensure they are drinking and taking their medication and also help them to go to the bathroom.

When the patient comes in the next morning, they tend to be completely calm and pain-free.

If the occlusive tapes were applied, you can remove them now and clean the face and see if any touch-up is needed if any wrinkles are still visible. Then apply the post-peel cream and the BSG powder to the face. You can also try to open the patient's eyes a bit and put a few eyedrops in them. This will help them to gradually open their eyes and for the lashes not to get stuck together.

Please reiterate to the patient that this powder must not come off for seven days and they are not allowed to wash it or wet it. Give them the remainder of the powder sachet and instruct them to powder their face a few times daily in the first two to three days to keep the powder dry with a yellow colour. Dark yellow or green means the powder is wet and needs to be topped up.

Hair washing is strictly not allowed for at least eight days. They may use a very small amount of Fucidin ointment if the skin cracks and becomes sore or bleeds a bit. It is only on day seven that they are supposed to cover the entire face with Bepanthen ointment and go to bed. Generally most of the crust will then easily come off on day eight.

During this week relative rest is necessary! Plenty of fluids and liquid food through a straw. Chewing is strictly not allowed. They must keep taking their medication daily as instructed.

With regards to follow-up appointments written in the consent form, I obviously adapt these according to each patient. The day one review is always compulsory. The day three review is preferably face-to-face, but if the patient lives far away and wants to recover at home, I am also happy with a virtual video consultation; and the same for day seven and day eight–nine reviews. Usually I will see the patient the day after the peel, then on day three, and then after the yellow crust has been removed. You can be flexible with the review dates, but day one and day three reviews are very important. We discuss all these reviews with the patient before the procedure and create as many quick follow-up visits as necessary.

Once the yellow crust comes off, the face will be very red and sometimes itchy but very smooth and still a bit swollen. It is a good idea to use Bepanthen ointment or a very thick sunblock on the first day or two as the skin will be very sensitive to use anything else. From day three they can usually tolerate their aftercare creams and sunblock and makeup.

Their skin will have some minor peeling for the next two weeks. After two weeks the skin looks pretty good except for the intense erythema. It may take several weeks before the erythema settles down. Usually around four to six months after the peel the full results can be appreciated as the neocollagenesis would have been completed by then. This would be a great time to see your patient again and take the after pictures and offer them further treatments such as a repeat of the botulinum toxin and, of course, skincare advice.

MOSAIC PEEL AFTERCARE

There is little difference between the aftercare for a mosaic peel and that for a full-face phenol peel. The only difference really is that the areas that were treated with TCA will not be covered by BSG powder and they will have sunscreen on them to protect them. I would recommend that the patient cleanses those areas only with a very gentle cleanser and cotton pads twice daily and reapplies the sunscreen. They must be very careful not to remove any of the BSG powder and keep topping it up, as previously explained.

Everything else is exactly as per full-face phenol peeling.

Please refer back to Chapter three to see all the aftercare forms.

REFERENCE

1. Deprez P, Full-face phenol: Postpeel care, in: *Textbook of chemical peels*, second edition, CRC Press, Boca Raton, 2016: 295–306.

Complications

12

Complications can occur even with the best technical abilities and the best aftercare; it just happens and we need to deal with them as they occur. The deeper a peel, the more risk of complications; however, even superficial peels can cause complications. We can generally avoid complications by sticking to the peel protocols and preparing the patient's skin very well and being strict with the aftercare (1,2).

There follow some of the complications that we may come across.

POOR OR INSUFFICIENT RESULT

Discussing the patient's expectations right from the onset will help prevent disappointment in the results. If your patient expects to look ten years younger after one single retinol peel, they will certainly be disappointed. Make sure you discuss options in detail and assess their expectations first.

Selecting the wrong peel type to achieve a specific result could also lead to disappointment. Equally, selecting the wrong patient for a peel could cause poor results too. For example, selecting a glycolic peel to remove deep peri-oral lines will lead to disappointment, or giving a patient with acne scarring a salicylic acid peel will lead to lack of improvement in the acne scarring.

Choosing the wrong peel depth will also lead to poor results. For example, performing a single superficial peel will not remove years of sun damage and deep wrinkles.

Insufficient skin preparation will usually always lead to a poor result or further complications, so it should be taken seriously. The thicker the skin or the oilier the skin is, the harder it is to penetrate, so better or longer skin preparation time and/or a deeper peel may be required to achieve results (Figure 12.1). One of the reasons why skin prep is important is to actually reduce the oil levels in the skin. When skin is relatively less oily, it will allow better penetration of any acid. For this reason the use of heavy moisturizers, including those based on mineral oil, is not a good idea as part of a peel prep routine.

A word of caution about deep phenol peels: phenol is not the answer to everything. Although it is a wonderful agent to deal with deep wrinkles and skin laxity, it performs less well in thick skin. Skin that is too thick or too sebaceous actually responds better to a combination of abrasion and TCA, as discussed previously.

DOI: 10.1201/9781003244134-12

187

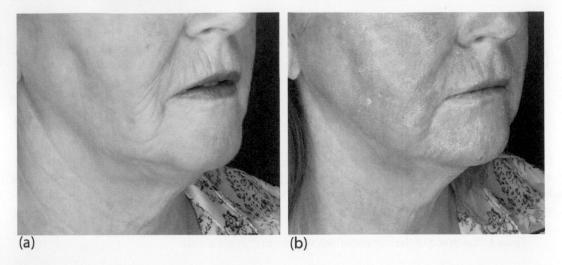

(a)   (b)

FIGURE 12.1 (a) Before and (b) eight days after a full-face 60% phenol peel with full occlusion. It is quite obvious that the upper lip lines have not fully been treated. This patient will need a touch up on the upper lip to try and eradicate those deeper lines. A repeat touch up phenol peel can be done on the upper lip only within a month without any risk of causing demarcation lines.

PROLONGED DOWNTIME

This could happen due to insufficient skin preparation. Well-prepared skin is in an active state and recovers far more quickly and with far fewer issues; well-prepared skin will recover five to six days after a medium TCA peel, whereas poorly prepped skin may take as long as two weeks to heal.

This could also happen due to the peel penetrating a bit deeper than expected, for example, by use of a strong retinoid for preparation too close to the actual peel date, or applying multiple coats of TCA in the same area.

Not following aftercare instructions at home could also cause prolonged downtime and issues further down the line. Perhaps restarting the active products too soon may result in irritation and prolonged erythema, or maybe the patient started using over-the-counter beauty products that may have caused irritation or an allergic reaction as the skin was more permeable and not fully recovered after the peel.

Active skincare products need to be reintroduced slowly after a peel in order to avoid this complication. Please always make sure that you include the post-peel aftercare products in the peel treatment so your patient has everything they need to use at home and are not left wondering what to do next.

POST-INFLAMMATORY HYPERPIGMENTATION (3)

Post-inflammatory hyperpigmentation (PIH) is very often due to lack of appropriate skin preparation and lack or insufficient use of tyrosinase inhibitors both before and after the peel. Obviously, lack of sun protection could cause this as well.

I have even had a patient who developed peri-orbital PIH after a mosaic peel with deep phenol in the peri-orbital region because they went and sat in the garden under the sun in the weeks immediately after their peel. So despite the fact that they had skin type II and did use sun protection, the phenol peel (which generally does not cause PIH) ended up having this issue. Fortunately, the problem was resolved within a few weeks of using tyrosinase inhibitors and sun protection.

Lack of patient compliance to both the prep phase and aftercare instructions is always an issue that could lead to PIH. Maybe they are using their SPF but perhaps not enough of it, or perhaps they are not avoiding the sun and exposing their face to bright sunlight. We can't be in control of what the patient does at home, but the more accurate we are with our instructions, the less likely it is that these types of issues will arise.

Choosing the wrong peel type for the wrong skin type can also be a cause; for example, a TCA peel on skin Fitzpatrick type IV without any skin prep is almost guaranteed to lead to PIH.

A peel penetrating too deep on darker skin types could lead to PIH, for example, a simple glycolic peel that was left on the skin too long or not properly neutralized on a dark skin type.

As discussed previously, PIH is treatable and if treated early on, it will most likely recover without any trace.

UNEVEN RESULT

Insufficient skin preparation may lead to the acid not being absorbed evenly over the entire surface of the skin. This could result in an uneven level of oiliness in the skin, which in turn will lead to an uneven penetration of the acid. This could also lead to an uneven level of tyrosinase inhibition in the skin and therefore cause dyschromia after the peel.

People are not always great at uniformly applying their products to the face. From experience I know that a lot of women focus the application of their products on the peri-oral area, especially the chin and sometimes the cheeks. So the full face gets an uneven level of treatment. The best way to apply a product to the face is to take out the full amount of any product that is required either on your fingertip or on the palm of your hand, and then to take small amounts of that product and apply it like dots all over the face, then blending the dots with the fingertips until the entire face is blended in.

Uneven application of the peel may also result in an uneven result. This is why it is important to divide the face into sections and treat each section methodically to avoid some areas getting too much and some too little application. If using, for example, TCA, the level of frosting will give us an idea of how far we have gone into the skin. What we use to apply the TCA with will obviously make a difference: for example, if we use cotton buds, we would get a different result compared to using a gauze swab. Also the pressure with which we apply the peel will make a difference; the harder we press, the more acid we push into the skin. Finally, the amount of acid on, for example, the cotton bud may vary per area of application, which will result in a different level of frosting. Because of all these possible variations, it is important that we try and standardize our procedure so that we make the peeling process as even as possible over the entire area.

PROLONGED ERYTHEMA

This is an expected side effect after a deep phenol peel, which needs to be discussed with the patient in detail during the consultation. Deep peels can cause erythema for up to three months, although in the majority of cases after six to eight weeks it becomes mild and not very noticeable.

Insufficient skin preparation and most importantly non-adherence to aftercare instructions could also cause this issue.

As mentioned previously, the use of active ingredients or over-the-counter cosmetics too soon after a peel can prolong or worsen erythema.

Please bear in mind that the use of retinoids both before and after the peel can cause longer erythema, but again this is an expected side effect and not a complication.

A very important fact to remember is that localized prolonged erythema could be an early sign of scarring, which is discussed further on.

REBOUND PIGMENTATION

This is very common when treating stubborn pigmentary disorders such as melasma. It is very often due to insufficient skin preparation or lack of use of appropriate tyrosinase inhibitors. Of course, lack of sun protection would have the same effect. Explaining this to your patient before the peel is extremely important.

Lack of aftercare or insufficient sun protection after the peel can most definitely be a cause. Most patients do not use enough sun protection and do not adhere to sun avoidance, so it is only logical that they will have a rebound of their pigmentation after the peel if they don't.

This can obviously be very disheartening for both the patient and the practitioner. Especially when treating melasma it is so important to really discuss this issue with the patient during the initial consultation and to document this. Melasma is very often not curable and will at some point come back. Using a good (prolonged) preparation phase and a solid aftercare/maintenance routine will give the best results with the least chance of any recurrence.

HERPES SIMPLEX (4)

The most common viral infection after a peel is of, course, herpes simplex.

If herpes simplex is present on the day of the peel, the procedure has to be postponed. It is an absolute contraindication to treat someone with an active herpetic lesion.

For those with a history of recurring herpes I would give them prophylactic antivirals, even for superficial peels.

I always give prophylactic antivirals for medium peels (five to seven days) and for deep peels (10–15 days). Herpes can create big problems if not prevented on skin that is recovering from a peel. It can literally erupt all over the face and cause pigmentation and scarring. It doesn't always occur on the lips either, but could be in any area of the face. (See Figure 12.2.)

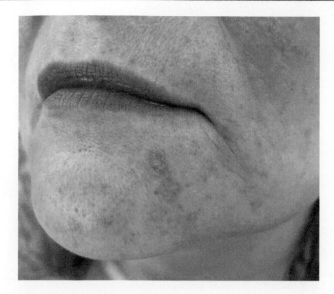

FIGURE 12.2   A small outbreak of herpes simplex at around ten days post-peel, which started around day three post-medium TCA peel on the chin. The patient was worried about this causing a scar but full recovery was achieved with a course of antiviral medication and aftercare creams.

BACTERIAL INFECTIONS (5)

Fortunately, bacterial infections are not very common in peels (Figure 12.3). Always bear in mind that impetigo could suddenly spread across large areas, so if in doubt always treat with antibiotics. For any mosaic peel or full-face deep peels, I always give seven days' worth of prophylactic antibiotics.

It is always important to have the same level of hygiene when performing peels as when doing injectable treatments. Make sure your hands are clean. Always wear gloves. Do not touch the patient's face without gloves. You are not performing a facial in a spa! Always cleanse thoroughly and make absolutely sure there is no makeup residue left on the face before the peel. Use clean instruments. Keep your trolley clean and tidy. Use sterile needles and syringes when drawing out acids from their vials.

Do not allow your patient to touch their face or apply any makeup immediately after the peel (sometimes you have to watch them like a hawk as this message does not seem to sink in with some patients, unfortunately).

Reiterate the aftercare instructions – when to wash the face, when to wash their hair, which creams to apply, using clean towels and pillow covers, staying away from animals and young children, etc.

Not everyone has the same basic level of understanding of hygiene – always remember that! So exaggerate the dos and don'ts and you have a better chance of avoiding infections. I recently had a patient who was worried about an infected lesion on the face a few days after a peel. When questioned she mentioned that her dog had been licking her aftercare cream off her face. When advised not to allow the dog to do that anymore, she replied 'she will try'.

For phenol peels, strict hygiene and strict adherence to the aftercare instructions is a must, especially in the first five days after the peel.

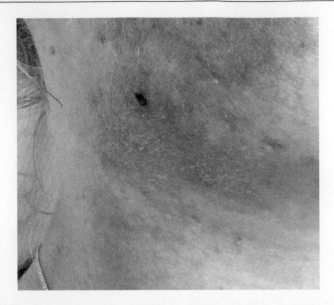

FIGURE 12.3   An example of bacterial infection; however, this was not after a peel. I have been fortunate enough to never see bacterial infection after any peels (yet). This was a patient who had a simple, very small lesion cautery on the jawline. A few days later she presented with this red rash extending over the cheek and going down the neck. This is very typical of skin bacterial infection and will need to be treated with a course of oral antibiotics.

SCARRING (6)

This is of course the scariest side effect of a chemical peel; fortunately, it is not very common.

It could occur due to insufficient skin preparation or to overly aggressive skin preparation – for example, using very strong retinoids for a prolonged period of time and not stopping them until right before a peel. This in itself could cause scarring even with a medium TCA peel, never mind a deep peel. So choosing the correct skin prep products is very important. Always look at the protocols given to you on your training session and do not deviate from them if you don't have the experience or expertise to do so.

It could also occur due to selecting the wrong patient – for example, offering a patient with a history of keloid scarring with Fitzpatrick skin type V a medium TCA peel without skin prep and really taking the peel to its maximum limit of depth. Or perhaps your patient is a carrier for a genetic disorder that affects their healing or collagen. This is a tough one and impossible to know if not previously diagnosed (see the list of contraindications in Chapter 4). Anyone with potentially delayed healing (for example, diabetes mellitus whether it is type one or two) should be treated with caution.

The issue could also arise from infections, as previously discussed. Infections can lead to scarring, and that's why it is so important to prevent them.

Finally, the application of the peel plays a role as well. Was the peel applied evenly? Did we insist on a specific area too much during the procedure? Did we apply too many coats in an area? Did we go too deep?

Again, try to stick to your protocols and deviate as little as possible to stay in the safety margins.

How to treat scarring:

The first step in treating scarring is spotting it early on and making sure it does not become a full-blown scar – hence the repeated after-peel visits after a deep peel. Scarring often starts as an area of excessive erythema that can feel a bit different in texture to the rest of the skin. We call it induration, so a bit thicker or harder to the touch. Or it could simply start as an area that is healing slower than other areas, so delayed re-epitheliazation could be a very early sign. If you suspect scarring, start treating it as soon as possible, and I would recommend you have weekly visits with the patient.

Treatment measures that can help are topical potent steroids, intralesional steroids, topical silicone application, LED therapy, and microneedling. I have found a combination approach to be most successful in case of early scar formation. I would generally recommend starting with immediate use of a potent steroid cream such as Betnovate twice daily. This helps very well to reduce the itching and discomfort that can often accompany early scarring. It should, however, be restricted to at maximum a couple of weeks and no longer. I also find simultaneously starting the patient on a silicone gel twice daily under the steroid cream helps a lot.

If you have access to LED light therapy, do use it; red light is great at speeding up the healing process and reducing erythema.

In my opinion if the scar does not seem to improve within two weeks, one should not hesitate to start using intralesional steroids. Once you start using intralesional steroids, it is advisable to stop the use of topical steroids but continue with all the other measures. You can use Triamcinolone for injection, but make sure you dilute it to inject the lesions very carefully and sparingly. Then review and possibly retreat in three to four weeks.

Gentle microneedling can also be used to soften the scars and to help to blend them in with the surrounding skin.

Any areas of delayed healing, prolonged erythema, prolonged itching, or areas with induration should be followed up carefully to stop scar formation. Early treatment will stop the scar from ever becoming obvious and will allow good healing and a great outcome (Figures 12.4 to 12.9).

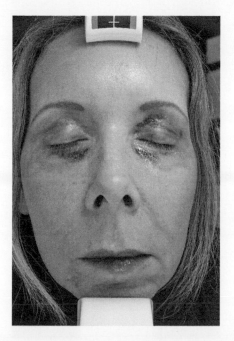

FIGURE 12.4 An example of a patient who had a mosaic peel on the peri-orbital area and ended up with delayed healing. This picture was taken on day 11 post-peel. At this stage one would expect complete re-epithialisation of the area with the expected erythema. However in this case the healing is taking too long. In such cases I would strongly recommend weekly visits to the clinic to continue monitoring the healing process and to start up treatments if necessary.

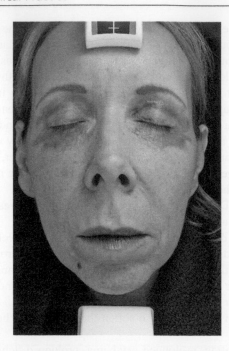

FIGURE 12.5 The same patient at week seven post-peel. The patient did develop hypertrophic scarring. The erythematous skin became hard and indurated. A course of intralesional Triamcinolone injections had to be commenced with topical silicone gel therapy and weekly LED red light sessions.

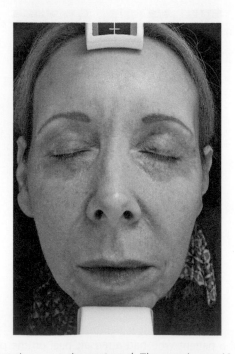

FIGURE 12.6 The same patient three months post-peel. The scarring and induration are definitely settling down and the erythema is finally dissipating. Further weekly aftercare will ensure a positive outcome for a complication that could have ended up very ugly if the patient had panicked and had become uncooperative.

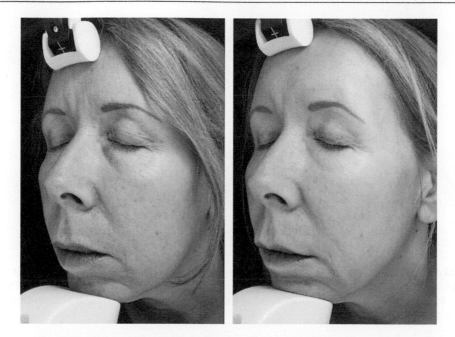

FIGURE 12.7 The same patient before and six months after the peel. The complication has been corrected, and the patient is very happy with the outcome and the level of skin resurfacing and tightening despite the slight hypopigmentation in the peri-orbital area. Further treatment of the face with tyrosinase inhibitors and/or a TCA peel will create a more blended even look.

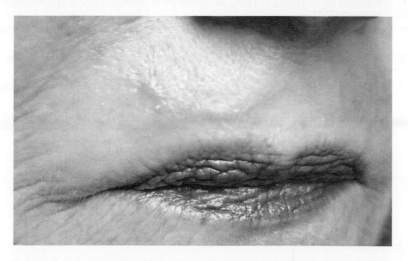

FIGURE 12.8 The top lip of a patient who had localized 60% phenol with occlusion on her top lip only. After roughly two months post-peel, this area of scarring started to appear out of nowhere. During those two months she had the usual erythema but did mention some itching on and off in that area.

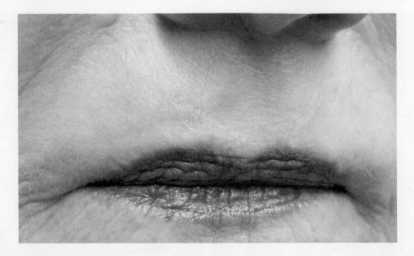

FIGURE 12.9   The same patient roughly ten months after this issue occurred. I treated the area with a few sessions of Triamcinolone intralesional injections. The result is not 100% perfect, but careful revisions and continued assessment and treatment can avoid scars from becoming true keloids and causing long term disfigurement.

REFERENCES

1. Deprez P, Alpha hydroxy acids: Side effects of AHAs, in: *Textbook of chemical peels*, second edition, CRC Press, Boca Raton, 2016: 63–64.
2. Deprez P, Complications of chemical peels, in: *Textbook of chemical peels*, second edition, CRC Press, Boca Raton, 2016: 325–373.
3. Deprez P, Treating melasma, chloasma and postinflammatory hyperpigmentation, in: *Textbook of chemical peels*, second edition, CRC Press, Boca Raton, 2016: 116–125.
4. Obagi ZE, Herpes simplex infection, in: *Obagi skin health restoration and rejuvenation*, Springer, New York, 2000: 230.
5. Obagi ZE, Bacterial infection, in: *Obagi skin health restoration and rejuvenation*, Springer, New York, 2000: 230–231.
6. Obagi ZE, Delayed, unanticipated reactions/true complications, hypertrophic reactions and keloids, in: *Obagi skin health restoration and rejuvenation*, CRC Press, Boca Raton, 2000: 240–242.

Conclusion

So you have come to the end of this book. I hope it was an enjoyable experience for you, and I hope I have been able to give you plenty of tips to safely perform your peels of choice.

Please remember this book or any textbook will never replace a training lecture with hands-on experience. Also start from the beginning and build up your experience. If you wanted to become an astronaut, you wouldn't start your career by doing a free walk in space; it would take you years of study, practice, and experience to do that, so why should anyone think we should be able to perform a full face deep peel if we have not even done a glycolic peel?

Please feel free to use the sample consent forms provided to create your own forms and adapt them to your practice. Paperwork can be boring, but it has to be done. Your patient has to read the forms, understand them, and agree to the treatment despite the potential complications. Always prepare your patient before the peel. The longer the prep phase, the better the results, the fewer the side effects, and the happier the patient experience.

I have found that it is best to include all the prep and aftercare products in the price of your peel treatment. This way your patient has everything they need. If required, I also include the price of any medication or investigations into the price as well. So the price you charge should reflect all these added extras.

If you have any questions about further hands-on training, please feel free to contact me.

Attending conferences and teaching sessions will help you to continuously keep your knowledge up to date and to keep up with the changes in this medical field. So never stop learning and never think you know it all.

Feel free to get yourself a detailed textbook on chemical peels such as the textbook written by Dr Philippe Deprez, which I have found to be an absolute must for my practice. This book will never replace the information that you will gain from a textbook, so use it as a practical guide to help you become familiar with the peeling processes.

I wish you all the best and look forward to seeing your successes.

Index

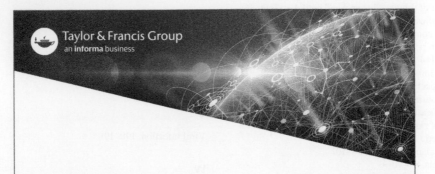

Printed and bound by CPI Group (UK) Ltd, Croydon, CR0 4YY

23/10/2024

01778379-0001